Understanding Kidney Diseases

Hugh Rayner • Mark Thomas • David Milford

Understanding Kidney Diseases

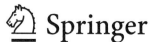 Springer

Hugh Rayner
Department of Renal Medicine
Birmingham Heartlands Hospital
Birmingham
UK

David Milford
Birmingham Children's Hospital
Birmingham
UK

Mark Thomas
Department of Renal Medicine
Birmingham Heartlands Hospital
Birmingham
UK

ISBN 978-3-319-23457-1   ISBN 978-3-319-23458-8   (eBook)
DOI 10.1007/978-3-319-23458-8

Library of Congress Control Number: 2015956618

Springer Cham Heidelberg New York Dordrecht London

Printed on acid-free paper

Springer International Publishing AG Switzerland is part of Springer Science+Business Media (www.springer.com)

We dedicate this book to people who live with kidney disease and the clinicians who care for them.

Foreword

Great teachers make their subjects appealing. Doctors Rayner, Thomas and Milford have certainly done that for renal science and kidney medicine. They have taken up-to-date molecular biology, physiology made complicated at medical school, innovative therapeutics and an intimate understanding of twenty-first century holistic healthcare, and molded a superb monograph accessible to students, vital for doctors in training and definitely of value for all practitioners of kidney care.

Kidney disease is common, harmful and treatable. Early detection, accurate diagnosis, systematic monitoring and evidence-based interventions are the key to improving outcomes. Doctor Rayner and colleagues bring their experience as front-line clinicians, researchers and educators to explain kidney problems clearly and concisely, simplifying where possible and highlighting areas of controversy or ambiguity where necessary.

Given the central role of the kidneys in maintaining the *milieu intérieur*, it is not surprising that kidney diseases provide a route to understanding a range of other metabolic, immunological and genetic conditions. This book balances clarity in describing these classic disorders with insights into the interaction between diseases in multimorbid patients. The compassion of the authors as practicing physicians is revealed in the excellent chapter on planning for transplantation or dialysis.

Those who have the pleasure of reading this book will gain a deep understanding of kidney diseases, knowledge of contemporary treatments and familiarity with systems to manage populations and personalise care. They will be better doctors and able to apply the lessons learned in whichever branch of medicine they practice.

Professor Donal O'Donoghue
President of the Renal Association
First NHS National Clinical Director for Kidney Care
Salford, UK

About the Authors

Dr. Hugh Rayner gained a first class degree in physiology at Cambridge University before qualifying with honours at the London Hospital Medical College in 1981. He was awarded an MD from the University of Leicester for studies on experimental models of kidney disease. After a number of training posts, including a year as clinical fellow in Melbourne, Australia, he was appointed as a consultant in renal and general medicine in Birmingham in 1993.

As part of his studies for the Diploma in Medical Education from Dundee University in 1996, he presented a dissertation on the interpretation of serum creatinine and published a consensus curriculum for undergraduate renal medicine [1]. He is a full-time nephrologist, clinical lead for the West Midlands Renal Network, and continues to teach renal medicine to undergraduates and trainee doctors.

Dr. Mark Thomas studied Biological Sciences and Medicine as an undergraduate at Kings College London and Westminster Medical School. After postgraduate training, he was a Research Fellow at Washington University Medical School in St Louis, USA, for 3 years, studying models of proteinuric renal disease. This interest continued during Senior Registrar training in Leicester. He has been a Consultant Nephrologist and Physician at the Heart of England Foundation Trust in Birmingham since 1998.

He has had a clinical research interest in acute kidney injury (AKI) for some years, including earlier detection and intervention in AKI. He is chief investigator for the Acute Kidney Outreach to Reduce Deterioration and Death (AKORDD) study, a large pilot study of AKI outreach. He has chaired clinical guideline development groups for AKI and anaemia management in CKD for the UK National Institute for Health and Care Excellence (NICE).

Dr. David Milford commenced basic paediatric training in 1983 and higher paediatric training at Sheffield Children's Hospital in 1986. He undertook research in the Department of Nephrology, Birmingham Children's Hospital, into the epidemiology of diarrhoea-associated haemolytic uraemic syndrome, resulting in several major publications and a thesis for Doctor of Medicine. He was appointed consultant nephrologist at Birmingham Children's Hospital in 1992. His interests include hypertension, acute kidney injury and renal transplantation.

Reference

1. Rayner HC. A model undergraduate core curriculum in adult renal medicine. Med Teacher. 1995;17:409–12.

Preface

This book provides you with the essential understanding you need to assess someone with kidney disease. The chapters follow the sequence taken during a consultation in a clinic or when clerking a patient. At each stage, we explain the principles and concepts underlying the things that make renal medicine seem difficult. We aim to answer those questions you may have been afraid to ask:

- What should I ask about and what tests should I order?
- How do I tell if kidney failure is acute or chronic?
- Are ACE inhibitors good or bad?

and many more.

Time is an important factor in kidney diseases. The same diagnosis can cause different symptoms and signs as the disease progresses over days, months, years and decades. It can be hard to make sense of one disease that can present in many different ways. To overcome this problem, we have included over 200 figures, including lots of graphs and charts. As Arthur Brisbane, the American newspaper editor said: "Use a picture. It's worth a thousand words".

The commonest chart is the graph of the eGFR (estimated glomerular filtration rate). This shows you how kidney function changes over time and helps you to make a diagnosis, decide when to do tests, monitor response to treatment, and plan dialysis and transplantation. And crucially, it shows the patient how they are getting on.

We have illustrated the book with case examples that are based upon patients we have cared for. Details have been altered to protect confidentiality and the patients have given written consent for information about them to be used. We hope their stories make the diseases more understandable and memorable, and that you will be stimulated to learn more about this fascinating subject.

We have included references to detailed reviews and original research studies if you wish to explore items in greater depth.

Birmingham, UK   Hugh Rayner
Birmingham, UK   Mark Thomas
Birmingham, UK   David Milford

Disclaimer

Although every effort is made to ensure that the information in this book is accurate, the ultimate responsibility for assessment and treatment of a patient rests with the practicing physician. Neither the publishers nor the authors can be held responsible for errors or for any consequences arising from the use of information contained herein.

Acknowledgements

We are indebted to the following for their contributions:

Roger Adkins, Colin Aldridge, Lise Bankir, Indy Dasgupta, Simon Dodds, Jo Ewing, John Evans, Agnes Fogo, Jonathan Freedman, Matthew Graham-Brown, Aarn Huissoon, Thirumala Krishna, Chris Lote, Thomas Mettang, Donal O'Donoghue, Michael Riste, Steve Smith, David Tudway, Es Will, Teun Wilmink, Chris Winearls.

Pathology images by Gerald Langman.

Clinical images by *mediahub agency*.

Additional artwork by Anthony Williams and Andrea Tibbitts.

Contents

1 Kidney Anatomy and Physiology   1
The Basis of Clinical Nephrology

The Anatomy of the Kidney.   1
Turning Blood into Urine.   1
Changes in Kidney Function over a Lifetime   5
References 10

2 Measuring Kidney Function 11
Quantifying Glomerular Filtration from Laboratory Tests

How Can Kidney Function Be Measured? 11
How Can GFR Be Estimated from Serum Creatinine? 13
Are These Estimates Accurate and Reliable? 15
Interpreting eGFR Values. 17
Not All Changes in Serum Creatinine Are Caused
by Changes in GFR 23
    Dietary Creatinine 24
    Changes in Muscle Mass. 25
    Tubular Secretion of Creatinine. 25
Serum Urea and Creatinine – Different Measures
of Kidney Function 26
References 28

3 Plot All the Dots 31
Graphs Reveal the Progression of Kidney Disease

Analysing Variation in eGFR. 34
Interpreting Variation in an eGFR Graph. 38
Acute Kidney Injury – Equilibrating Creatinine 42
Dealing with Missing Data 44
Acute-On-Chronic Kidney Disease – Time in Two Dimensions. 45
References 48

xvii

4 How Are You Feeling?   51
The Symptoms of Uraemia

Stages of CKD   51
Uraemia and the Nervous System   52
References   57

5 Do You Have Any Long-Term Health Conditions?   59
Kidney Involvement in Multisystem Diseases

Diabetes Mellitus   59
Atherosclerosis   67
    Renal Artery Stenosis   67
    Cholesterol Crystal Embolisation (Atheroembolic Disease)   71
Chronic Infection and Inflammation   73
References   74

6 Are You Pregnant or Planning a Pregnancy?   77
How Pregnancy Affects the Kidneys and Vice Versa

Risks to the Baby   77
Risks to the Mother   77
Pre-Eclampsia   79
References   81

7 What Is Your Family History?   83
The Molecular Genetics of Inherited Kidney Diseases

The Glomerular Filtration Barrier   84
    Alport Syndrome   84
    Congenital Nephrotic Syndrome   84
The Tubules   86
    The Proximal Tubule   86
    The Loop of Henle   86
    The Distal Tubule   87
    The Collecting Duct   89
Uromodulin   90
Cystic Kidney Diseases   91
Kidney Tumours   94
The Lower Urinary Tract   95
References   99

8 What Have You Been Taking?   103
Nephrotoxicity from Medications and Other Chemicals

Vasoactive Drugs   103
    ACE inhibitors and Angiotensin Receptor Blockers   104
    Non-steroidal Anti-inflammatory Drugs   107
    Calcineurin Inhibitors – Two Sides of a Coin   108
    Mixing Vasoactive Drugs to Make MINT Cocktails   108

Tubulotoxic Drugs   110
    Lithium   110
    Aminoglycoside Antibiotics – Gentamicin   112
Interstitial Nephritis   112
Metformin – Villain or Victim?   112
Kidney Diseases Due to Toxins   113
    Cocaine and Heroin   113
    Mushroom Poisoning   114
    Chemical Poisoning   114
References   114

9 Height and Weight   117
   The Effects of Kidney Disease on Body Size and Composition

   Growing Up with Kidney Disease   117
   Transitional Care   123
   Obesity and Risk   123
   References   123

10 Blood Pressure   125
   A Common Theme in Kidney Disease

   Diurnal Variation in Blood Pressure   126
   Controlling Blood Pressure – Key to Preserving Kidney Function   129
   References   131

11 Test the Urine   133
   Understanding Haematuria, Proteinuria and Urinary Infection

   Haematuria   134
       How Red Cells Cross the Glomerular Filtration Barrier   135
       The Clinical Significance of Haematuria   136
   Myoglobinuria   142
   Proteinuria   143
   Nephrotic Syndrome   149
   Urine Infection   152
   References   158

12 Examine the Patient   161
   Physical Signs Related to Kidney Diseases

   Fluid Balance   161
       How Salt and Water Is Distributed in the Body   161
       How Excess Salt and Water Can Be Removed   163
   Assessing Fluid Balance in Acutely Ill Patients   164
   Physical Signs of Kidney Disease   167
   Examine the Abdomen   170
   References   171

13 **Full Blood Count, Urea and Electrolytes,**
    Bicarbonate, Bone Profile 173
    Laboratory Results and Kidney Diseases

    Anaemia.. 173
        Erythropoietin and the Regulation of Haemoglobin 173
        Why in the Kidneys?....................................... 175
        Kidney Disease Linked to Causes of Anaemia 176
    Acid, Base, Bicarbonate and Total CO_2......................... 180
    Vitamin D, Minerals, Bones and Blood Vessels 181
        Why is Vitamin D Activated in the Kidneys? 184
        Hyperparathyroidism....................................... 184
        Parathyroidectomy.. 186
        Hypercalcaemia.. 189
    References 194

14 **Immunology** 197
    Serological Tests That Help Diagnose Kidney Diseases

    Do the Right Test on the Right Patient......................... 197
    Immunoglobulins, Protein Electrophoresis, Free Light
    Chains in Serum and Urine 198
        Multiple Myeloma... 199
        Amyloidosis... 200
    Anti-nuclear Antibody, Anti-dsDNA Antibody 202
    Complement C3 and C4... 202
    Anti-streptolysin O (ASO) and Anti-DNAse B Antibodies............ 204
    Anti-neutrophil Cytoplasmic Antibody (ANCA)..................... 204
    Anti-glomerular Basement Membrane Antibody (Anti-GBM ab)........ 210
    Anti-phospholipase A_2 Receptor Antibody (Anti-PLA$_2$R ab) 211
    References 213

15 **Image the Urinary Tract** 215
    Strengths and Weaknesses of Different Radiology Modalities

    Ultrasound 215
        Appearances in Kidney Disease 215
        Urinary Tract Obstruction 220
    Isotope Renography... 223
    Computed Tomography 226
    The Risks and Benefits of Using Contrast Media 227
    References 229

16 **Should We Do a Kidney Biopsy?** 231
    Balancing the Diagnostic Benefits Against the Clinical Risks

    'Primum Non Nocere' – First, Do No Harm 231
    Is It Diabetic Nephropathy?................................... 232
    References 236

17 Make a Plan 237
When and How to Prepare for End-Stage Kidney Disease

Understanding Risk and Predicting the Future 237
Competing Risks: Dialysis or Death? 240
Prognostication: "Be Prepared" 241
Writing Letters to Patients 248
Choosing Treatment: Transplant, Haemodialysis,
Peritoneal Dialysis or No Dialysis? 249
When Should Dialysis Be Started? 249
Care of the Whole Person 250
References 251

18 Renal Replacement Therapy 255
Common Problems in Dialysis and Transplant Patients

Haemodialysis 255
Vascular Access 255
Complications of a Haemodialysis Catheter 262
Peritoneal Dialysis 262
Fluid Balance in a Dialysis Patient 263
Kidney Transplant 265
Causes of a Decline in Transplant Function 266
Infection 267
Malignancy 269
References 273

19 Epilogue 275
Scaling-Up Kidney Care from One Individual to a Whole Population

References 277

Multiple Choice Questions 279

Multiple Choice Question Answers 289

Index of Case Reports 291

Index of Histopathology, Radiology and Clinical Images 293

Index 295

Chapter 1
Kidney Anatomy and Physiology

The Basis of Clinical Nephrology

Abstract In this chapter we explain:
- The basic anatomy and physiology of the kidney
- How kidney function changes through life

The Anatomy of the Kidney

The kidneys are complex and beautiful organs. Their internal structure is revealed by anatomical studies using light and electron microscopy (Figs. 1.1, 1.2, 1.3, 1.4 and 1.5).

Turning Blood into Urine

The kidneys are central to homeostasis [2]. Through exquisite sensory mechanisms [3] they regulate blood pressure, water [4], sodium [5], potassium [6], acidity [7], bone minerals [8], and haemoglobin. But their core function is the excretion of the waste products of metabolism in urine.

About 22 % of cardiac output goes to the kidneys and about 20 % of the plasma is filtered, producing about 170 L of glomerular filtrate per day. Ninety-nine percent of this is reabsorbed as it flows along the nephrons so only about 1.5 L of urine is produced per day.

Filtration occurs through the glomerular filtration barrier [9]. This is made up of five layers [10] (Fig. 1.6):

- the glycocalyx covering the surface of the endothelial cells
- holes (fenestrations) in the glomerular endothelial cells
- the glomerular basement membrane
- the slit diaphragm between the foot-processes of the podocytes
- the sub-podocyte space between the slit diaphragm and the podocyte cell body

© Springer International Publishing Switzerland 2016
H. Rayner et al., *Understanding Kidney Diseases*,
DOI 10.1007/978-3-319-23458-8_1

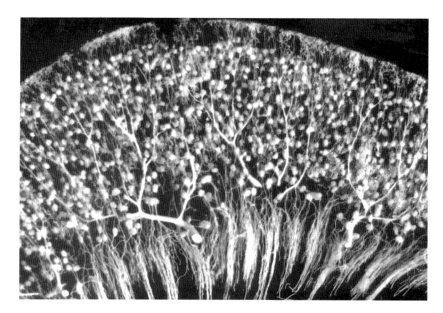

Fig. 1.1 Longitudinal section through the cortex and outer medulla of a rabbit kidney in which the artery has been injected with white Microfil. Microfil has filled the arteries, arterioles, glomerular tufts and the early part of the post-glomerular capillaries in the cortex and outer medulla (Courtesy of Dr Lise Bankir, Centre de Recherche des Cordeliers, Paris, France)

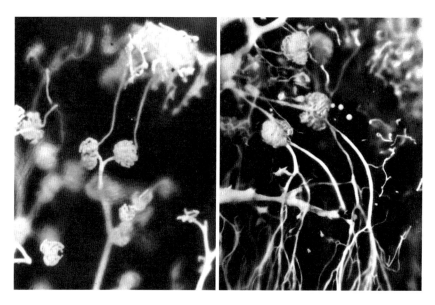

Fig. 1.2 Rabbit kidney injected with white Microfil through the renal artery. *Left*: detail of a longitudinal section showing a small part of the superficial cortex. The glomerular tufts of two superficial glomeruli are visible with their post-glomerular capillaries located in the very superficial cortex. *Right*: detail of a longitudinal section showing part of the deep cortex and the outer stripe of the outer medulla. The glomerular tufts of two juxtamedullary glomeruli are visible with their efferent arterioles that run towards the outer medulla where they give rise to vascular bundles (Courtesy of Dr Lise Bankir, Centre de Recherche des Cordeliers, Paris, France)

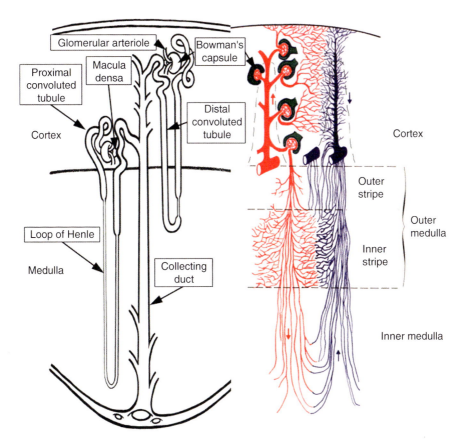

Fig. 1.3 Nephons and their blood supply. *Left*: a short looped- and a long looped-nephron. *Right*: the different vascular territories and their location in the four renal zones. For clarity, the cortex has been widened and the inner medulla compressed

The composition of glomerular filtrate is determined by the structure, arrangement and electrical charge of the collagen protein molecules that form the filtration barrier. So glomerular filtration is both size-selective and charge-selective; molecules that are too large or too highly charged cannot get through.

A substantial amount of albumin does get through the barrier, between 3.3 and 5.7 g per day. A proportion passes from the sub-podocyte space through the podocytes by transcytosis [11]. Passage of albumin through the barrier is increased by angiotensin II. Almost all the filtered albumin is reabsorbed by active uptake into the proximal tubular cells [12].

A simple model of the haemodynamics of glomerular filtration can be made from a garden hose (Fig. 1.7).

Glomerular filtration is held constant over a wide range of systemic and renal artery pressures by a process called autoregulation. Constriction and dilatation of the afferent arteriole is controlled by the macula densa, which is adjacent to the glomerulus. The macula densa senses the flow of sodium chloride through the tubule next to it. When this flow is increased, the macula densa causes constriction of the afferent arteriole to reduce the glomerular filtration rate.

Conversely, if the pressure of blood flowing into the kidney falls, the resistance in the afferent arteriole is reduced to maintain the pressure within the glomerulus. If the inflow pressure continues to drop, the efferent arteriole constricts under the influence of angiotensin II. This maintains the filtration pressure within the glomerulus. In our simple model (Fig. 1.7) pressing on the end of the hose represents the effect of angiotensin II, increasing the resistance to flow of blood out of the glomerulus via the efferent arteriole.

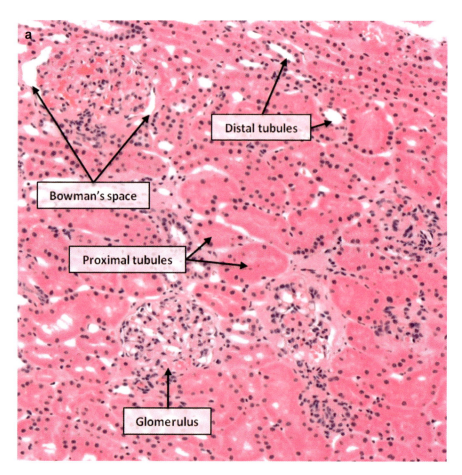

Figs. 1.4 (**a, b**) Light micrographs of normal renal cortex with the main structures indicated. Haematoxylin and eosin; **a** ×100, **b** ×200

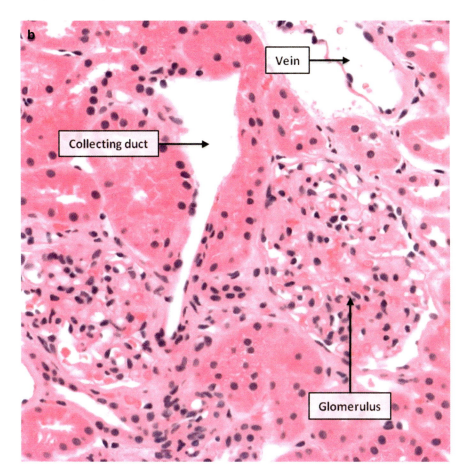

Fig. 1.4 (continued)

Changes in Kidney Function over a Lifetime

In the uterus, only about 2 % of cardiac output goes to the kidneys. Excretion of waste products produced by the foetus is via the placenta. Renal blood flow increases rapidly in the first week after birth as flow in the aorta increases and renal vascular resistance falls. By 1 month of age it has doubled and by 1 year it has reached adult levels in proportion to body size. Similarly, glomerular filtration rate (GFR) is about 10 % of the adult value at birth, rises rapidly in the first month and reaches adult levels by 1 year of age (see Fig. 1.8).

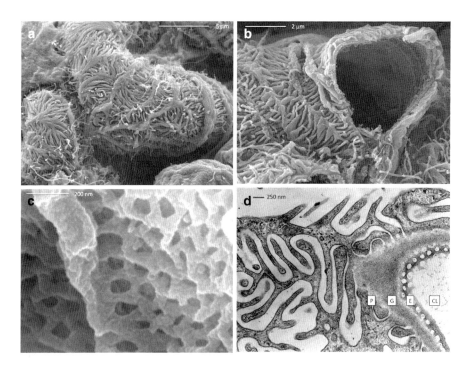

Fig. 1.5 Scanning electron micrographs of a mouse glomerular capillary. (**a**) The surface of a capillary showing podocyte (5000× by SecretDisc). (**b**) A cut open capillary revealing the endothelial lining (10,000× by SecretDisc). (**c**) The inner surface showing fenestrations in the endothelial cells (100,000× by SecretDisc). (**d**) Transmission electron micrograph of a section of glomerular capillary wall showing the layers that form the glomerular filtration barrier. *CL* capillary lumen, *E* endothelial cell fenestrations, *G* glomerular basement membrane, *P* podocyte slit diaphragm (Image **d** made available by James D. Jamieson and the Department of Cell Biology, Yale University School of Medicine. Original 3.25 in.×4 in. lantern slides were scanned at 600 dpi. Original magnification ×16,000. The original work has been cropped and modified with labels) [1]

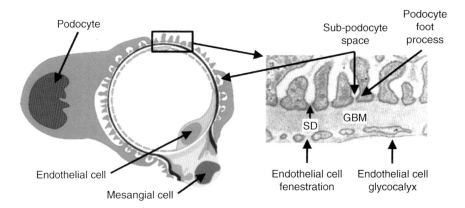

Fig. 1.6 The cells and five structural components that form the glomerular filtration barrier. *SD* slit diaphragm, *GBM* glomerular basement membrane

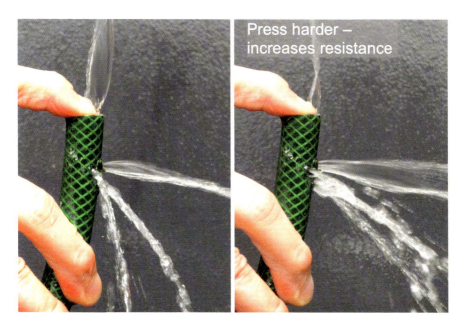

Fig. 1.7 The hose from the tap represents the afferent arteriole. Holes have been made near the end of the hose to represent fenestrations in the glomerular capillary wall. Pressing the finger on the end of the hose increases resistance in the efferent arteriole. This increases glomerular filtration pressure and flow rate

There is huge variation between people in the number of glomeruli per kidney. The average is approximately 800,000 but numbers can vary nine fold from approximately 200,000 to 1,800,000 [14].

There is less variation between people in GFR because the size and filtration rate per glomerulus increases as the number of glomeruli decreases. On average glomeruli are twice as big in people with the fewest compared to those with the most. Enlarged glomeruli are a feature of low birth weight, massive obesity, hypertension and cardiovascular disease, and are a sign of an increased risk of chronic kidney disease [15].

After the age of about 45 years there is a steady decline in the number of functioning nephrons as glomeruli undergo sclerosis. This is reflected in a decline in kidney blood flow and GFR (see Fig. 1.9). In males at age 40 years the mean kidney blood flow is 600 mL/min/1.73 m^2 and GFR is 120 mL/min/1.73 m^2. By age 80 years these have reduced to 300 and 70 mL/min/1.73 m^2 respectively [16]. Values for females are similar.

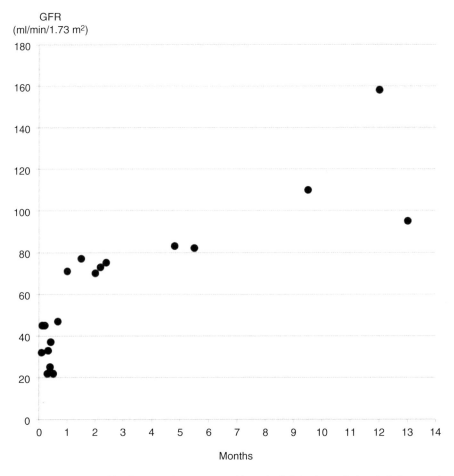

Fig. 1.8 Glomerular filtration rate (GFR) measured by a single injection technique in infants aged up to 13 months (Redrawn using data from Aperia et al. [13])

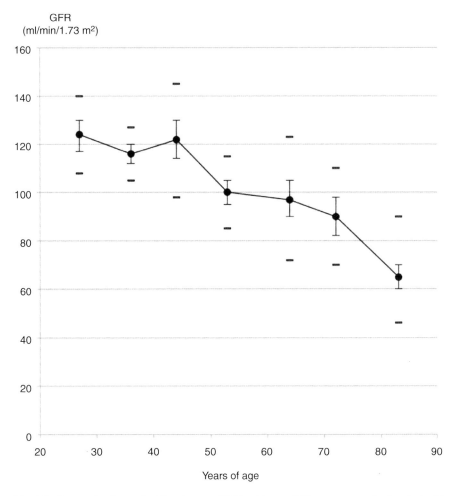

Fig. 1.9 Changes in glomerular filtration rate (GFR) with age. GFR was measured using the 'gold standard' inulin clearance method in 75 healthy males. *Error bars* indicate standard deviation of the mean. Outer lines indicate standard deviation of the distribution (Redrawn from [16])

References

1. Farquhar M.G, Wissig SL and Palade GE. Glomerular permeability. J Exp Med. 1961;113: 47–66. http://www.cellimagelibrary.org/images/37178.
2. Hoenig MP, Zeidel ML. Homeostasis, the milieu intérieur, and the wisdom of the nephron. Clin J Am Soc Nephrol. 2014;9(7):1272–81. doi:10.2215/CJN.08860813. http://cjasn.asnjournals.org/content/9/7/1272.full.
3. Pluznick JL, Caplan MJ. Chemical and physical sensors in the regulation of renal function. Clin J Am Soc Nephrol. pii: CJN.00730114. doi:10.2215/CJN.00730114. http://cjasn.asnjournals.org/content/early/2014/10/02/CJN.00730114.full.
4. Danziger J, Zeidel ML. Osmotic homeostasis. Clin J Am Soc Nephrol. CJN.10741013. doi:10.2215/CJN.10741013. http://cjasn.asnjournals.org/content/early/2015/03/30/CJN.10741013.full.
5. Palmer LG, Schnermann J. Integrated control of Na transport along the nephron. Clin J Am Soc Nephrol. CJN.12391213. doi:10.2215/CJN.12391213. http://cjasn.asnjournals.org/content/early/2014/08/05/CJN.12391213.full.
6. Subramanya AR, Ellison DH. Distal convoluted tubule. Clin J Am Soc Nephrol. 2014;9(12): 2147–63. doi:10.2215/CJN.05920613. http://cjasn.asnjournals.org/content/9/12/2147.full.
7. Curthoys NP, Moe OW. Proximal tubule function and response to acidosis. Clin J Am Soc Nephrol. 2014;9(9):1627–38. doi:10.2215/CJN.10391012. http://cjasn.asnjournals.org/content/9/9/1627.full.
8. Blaine J, Chonchol M, Levi M. Renal control of calcium, phosphate, and magnesium homeostasis. Clin J Am Soc Nephrol. CJN.09750913. doi:10.2215/CJN.09750913. http://cjasn.asnjournals.org/content/early/2014/11/30/CJN.09750913.full.
9. Pollak MR, Quaggin SE, Hoenig MP, Dworkin LD. The glomerulus: the sphere of influence. Clin J Am Soc Nephrol. 2014;9(8):1461–9. doi:10.2215/CJN.09400913. http://cjasn.asnjournals.org/content/9/8/1461.full.
10. Arkill KP, Qvortrup K, Starborg T, Mantell JM, Knupp C, Michel CC, Harper SJ, Salmon AHJ, Squire JM, Bates DO, Neal CR. Resolution of the three dimensional structure of components of the glomerular filtration barrier. BMC Nephrol. 2014;15:24. doi:10.1186/1471-2369-15-24. http://link.springer.com/article/10.1186/1471-2369-15-24/fulltext.html.
11. Schießl IM, Hammer A, Kattler V, Gess B, Theilig F, Witzgall R, Castrop H. Intravital imaging reveals angiotensin II–induced transcytosis of albumin by podocytes. J Am Soc Nephrol. pii: ASN.2014111125; published ahead of print June 26, 2015. doi:10.1681/ASN.2014111125. http://jasn.asnjournals.org/content/early/2015/06/25/ASN.2014111125.abstract.
12. Gekle M. Renal tubule albumin transport. Annu Rev Physiol. 2005;67:573–94. http://www.annualreviews.org/doi/abs/10.1146/annurev.physiol.67.031103.154845.
13. Aperia A, Broberger O, Thodenius K, Zetterström R. Development of renal control of salt and fluid homeostasis during the first year of life. Acta Paediatr Scand. 1975;64:393–8. http://onlinelibrary.wiley.com/doi/10.1111/j.1651-2227.1975.tb03853.x/abstract.
14. Hoy WE, Douglas-Denton RN, Hughson MD, Cass A, Johnson K, Bertram JF. A stereological study of glomerular number and volume: preliminary findings in a multiracial study of kidneys at autopsy. Kidney Int. 2003;63:S31–7. doi:10.1046/j.1523-1755.63.s83.8.x. http://www.nature.com/ki/journal/v63/n83s/full/4493733a.html.
15. Hoy WE, Hughson MD, Diouf B, Zimanyi M, Samuel T, McNamara BJ, Douglas-Denton RN, Holden L, Mott SA, Bertram JF. Distribution of volumes of individual glomeruli in kidneys at autopsy: association with physical and clinical characteristics and with ethnic group. Am J Nephrol. 2011;33 Suppl 1:15–20. doi:10.1159/000327044. Epub 2011 Jun 10. http://www.karger.com/Article/FullText/327044.
16. Davies DF, Shock NW. Age changes in glomerular filtration rate, effective renal plasma flow, and tubular excretory capacity in adult males. J Clin Invest. 1950;29(5):496–507. doi:10.1172/JCI102286. PMCID: PMC436086. http://www.jci.org/articles/view/102286.

Chapter 2
Measuring Kidney Function

Quantifying Glomerular Filtration from Laboratory Tests

Abstract In this chapter we explain:

- How serum creatinine is related to glomerular filtration rate (GFR)
- The limitations of creatinine as a measure of GFR
- How GFR is estimated from serum creatinine and cystatin C
- Common errors made when using eGFR
- How to interpret urea and creatinine together

How Can Kidney Function Be Measured?

To assess someone's kidney function, one would really like to measure their glomerular filtration rate (GFR). This can be done using a radioisotope tracer that is cleared from the blood solely by glomerular filtration, such as Cr-51 EDTA or Tc-99m DTPA. This technique is useful for research and when precise measurements of GFR are required. But it is impractical for routine repeated measurements.

Instead of measuring the clearance of an artificial tracer, routine assessment of kidney function uses the concentration of a substance produced by the body, creatinine, urea or cystatin C. Their concentration is determined by the balance between the rate of production and the rate of excretion.

When production and excretion have been stable for more than 24 h, an equilibrium concentration is reached. In equilibrium, the concentration is not affected by the volume of body water in which the substance is dissolved. Patients who are chronically fluid overloaded do not have a lower concentration due to dilution. The higher concentration found with dehydration is due to reduced kidney function, not haemoconcentration.

Creatinine would be the ideal choice for measuring kidney function if it was produced at a constant rate, freely filtered by the glomeruli, and neither reabsorbed nor secreted by the tubules. Unfortunately, it does not pass all these tests.

Creatinine is released into the bloodstream at a fairly constant rate from the breakdown of creatine in healthy skeletal muscles and is freely filtered by the glomeruli. In addition, 10–20 % of normal total creatinine excretion is by secretion into the tubules. As GFR declines that proportion increases and so serum creatinine does

© Springer International Publishing Switzerland 2016   11
H. Rayner et al., *Understanding Kidney Diseases*,
DOI 10.1007/978-3-319-23458-8_2

not increase as much as predicted from filtration. This is shown by comparing simultaneous measurements of serum creatinine and GFR using the gold standard inulin clearance technique (see Fig. 2.1).

The curved relationship between creatinine and GFR makes changes in serum creatinine hard to interpret correctly. Figure 2.2 shows a graph of serum creatinine against time in a man with declining kidney function. The shape of the line suggests that the rate of loss of kidney function accelerates over the years.

If we now add in GFR values, it is clear that kidney function has actually declined at a constant rate over the whole period (see Fig. 2.3).

Because of the inverse curved relationship between GFR and creatinine, the drop in GFR from 116 to 60 during the first 5 years causes a smaller increase in serum creatinine than the decline from 60 to 30 over the next 3 years.

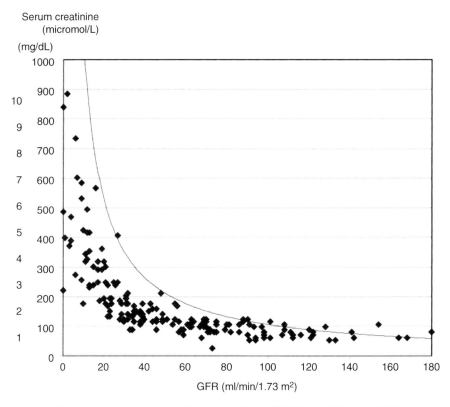

Fig. 2.1 Simultaneous measurements of serum creatinine (*filled diagonal box*) and GFR by inulin clearance in over 100 individuals. The *continuous line* represents the relationship between serum creatinine and GFR that would be found if creatinine was only filtered by glomeruli and not modified by the tubules (Redrawn from Shemesh et al. [1]).

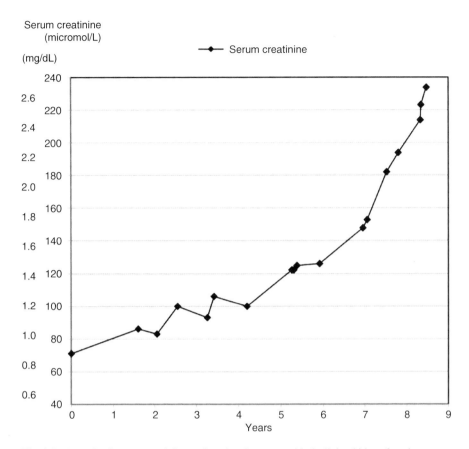

Fig. 2.2 A graph of serum creatinine against time in a man with declining kidney function

How Can GFR Be Estimated from Serum Creatinine?

To make serum creatinine results easy to interpret we need to convert them into estimates of the GFR (eGFR). Equations to do the conversion have been derived from databases containing simultaneous measurements of GFR, by a radioisotope clearance technique, and serum creatinine concentration. The four-variable MDRD equation was derived from measurements performed on adult patients with chronic kidney disease in the Modification of Diet in Renal Disease (MDRD) study [2].

eGFR values are standardised to a body surface area of 1.73 m^2 and so their calculation does not require the patient's body weight. This makes it possible for the laboratory to provide eGFR values automatically from the patient's age and sex.

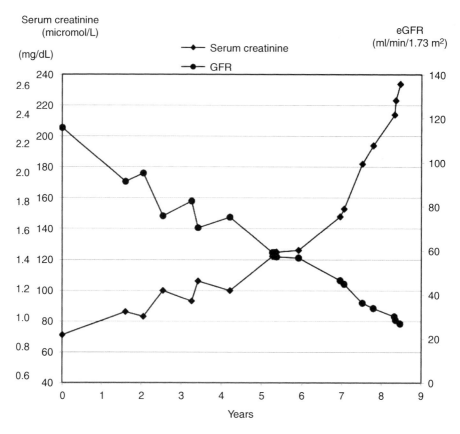

Fig. 2.3 A graph of serum creatinine and GFR against time in the same man as in Fig. 2.2

As the laboratory does not usually have reliable information about ethnicity, the adjustment for Afro-Caribbean race is done manually.

For children, different equations are available [3]. The commonest used is the Schwarz equation [4].

The Schwarz Equation [4]

$$\text{GFR}(\text{ml / min/ } 1.73 \text{ m}^2) = (0.413 \times \text{Height in cm} \times 88.4)$$
$$/\text{Creatinine in micromol / L}$$

$$\text{GFR}(\text{ml / min/ } 1.73 \text{ m}^2) = (0.413 \times \text{Height in cm}) / \text{Creatinine in mg / dL}$$

$$\text{GFR}(\text{ml / min/ } 1.73 \text{ m}^2) = 175 \times (\text{Creat})^{-1.154} \times (\text{Age})^{-0.203}$$
$$\times (0.742 \text{ if female}) \times (1.212 \text{ if black race})$$

This equation uses serum creatinine values calibrated against isotope dilution mass spectrometry (IDMS).

Are These Estimates Accurate and Reliable?

The 90 % confidence intervals of the estimates are wide. Using the MDRD equation, 90 % of estimates are within 30 % of the directly measured GFR and 98 % within 50 %. In children using the Schwarz equation, 80 % of estimates are within 30 % of the measured GFR. The estimates are less accurate in people with very abnormal body composition, such as amputees and malnourished patients.

The MDRD equation was derived from patients known to have kidney disease and a raised serum creatinine. It is inaccurate for estimating GFR from serum creatinine values in the normal range, i.e. outside the dataset used to derive the formula, for example in pregnancy [5]. The eGFR is not appropriate for situations in which a more accurate measurement of GFR is required, such as in the assessment of a potential transplant donor.

Because the MDRD equation underestimates the true GFR when serum creatinine values are in the normal range, people are at risk of being labelled as having kidney disease based upon these estimates. To reduce this, guidelines recommend that laboratories use the more recently developed CKD-EPI equations [6]. CKD-EPI gives estimates that are closer to the measured GFR at lower levels of serum creatinine, applying a different equation when creatinine is in the normal range [7, 8].

It is best to use the eGFR estimate provided by the laboratory that analysed the blood sample as that will include appropriate adjustments for the creatinine assay.

The accuracy of GFR estimates is less relevant when they are used to follow an individual patient over time. Here it is the shape of the graph rather than the exact value that is of interest. There is a good correlation between the slopes of measured and estimated GFR values over time. Also, patient-related factors affect the measured and estimated GFR slopes in a similar way, so slopes can be compared between patients [9, 10].

One way to validate the use of eGFR graphs is to compare them with graphs of measured GFR in patients with similar pathological processes. Figure 2.4 shows sequential measurements of GFR from five patients with autosomal dominant polycystic kidney disease (ADPKD). The trajectory of GFR is linear, although the gradient varies between patients.

The CKD-EPI Equations [7]

Black
Female

Serum creatinine

$\leq 62 \ \mu mol\,/\,L\left(\leq 0.7 \ mg\,/\,dL\right)$ $GFR = 166 \times \left(Scr\,/\,0.7\right)^{-0.329} \times \left(0.993\right)^{Age}$

$> 62 \mu mol\,/\,L\left(> 0.7 \ mg\,/\,dL\right)$ $GFR = 166 \times \left(Scr\,/\,0.7\right)^{-1.209} \times \left(0.993\right)^{Age}$

Male

$$\le 80(\le 0.9) \quad GFR = 163 \times (Scr / 0.9)^{-0.411} \times (0.993)^{Age}$$

$$> 80(> 0.9) \quad GFR = 163 \times (Scr / 0.9)^{-1.209} \times (0.993)^{Age}$$

White or other ethnicity
Female

$$\le 62(\le 0.7) \quad GFR = 144 \times (Scr / 0.7)^{-0.329} \times (0.993)^{Age}$$

$$> 62(> 0.7) \quad GFR = 144 \times (Scr / 0.7)^{-1.209} \times (0.993)^{Age}$$

Male

$$\le 80(\le 0.9) \quad GFR = 141 \times (Scr / 0.9)^{-0.411} \times (0.993)^{Age}$$

$$> 80(> 0.9) \quad GFR = 141 \times (Scr / 0.9)^{-1.209} \times (0.993)^{Age}$$

CKD-EPI = Chronic Kidney Disease Epidemiology Collaboration
Scr = serum creatinine in mg/dL (micromol/L/88.4)
Age in years for ≥ 18

Graphs of estimated GFR from patients with ADPKD also have linear trajectories (see Fig. 2.5).

Interpreting eGFR Values

eGFR equations for men and women are different because, on average, men contain proportionately more muscle than women. Body composition also changes with age, the proportion of muscle declining as people grow older. Including these factors, we can draw a family of graphs of estimated GFR versus serum creatinine (see Fig. 2.6).

Females have a lower eGFR than males for any given serum creatinine value (see Fig. 2.7).

To derive the correct eGFR, the laboratory must be provided with the correct sex and date of birth. Using an incorrect adjustment causes a significant error in the

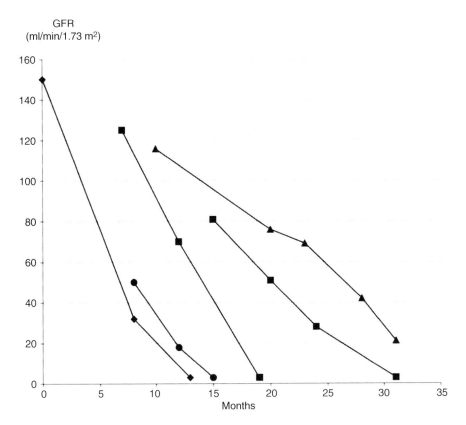

Fig. 2.4 Measurements of GFR using inulin or Cr-EDTA clearance from five patients with autosomal dominant polycystic kidney disease (ADPKD). The rate of decline is more rapid than found in most patients with ADPKD [11]

estimate, giving either false alarm or false reassurance, as shown by the following cases (Patients 2.1 and 2.2).

Patients with family names that are also used as first names are at particular risk of being labelled with the wrong sex (Patient 2.2).

The estimated GFR needs to be adjusted for Afro-Caribbean race but not for other ethnicities (see Fig. 2.10). This is because of genetically determined differences in skeletal muscle between racial groups. Compared to white Caucasians, black African people have 30–40 % higher activities of a number of enzymes involved in phosphagenic metabolic pathways, including creatine kinase [12].

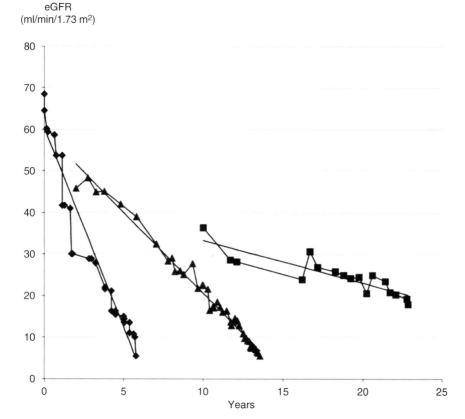

Fig. 2.5 eGFR graphs from three patients with ADPKD, chosen to show the wide variation in the eGFR gradient between patients

eGFR
(ml/min/1.73 m^2)

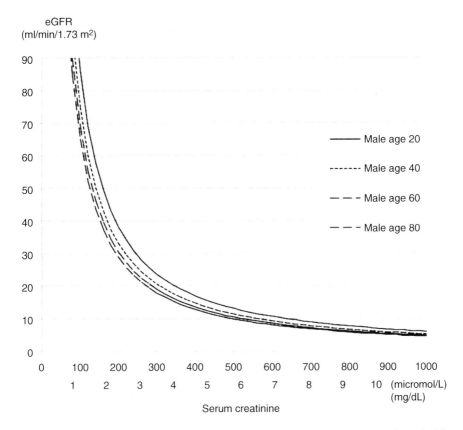

Fig. 2.6 A family of graphs of eGFR against serum creatinine, showing how the estimated GFR falls with age (MDRD equation)

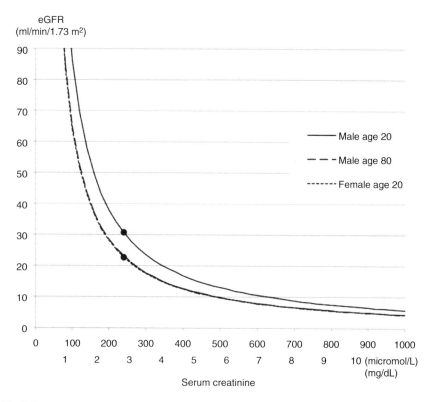

Fig. 2.7 eGFR calculated for a female aged 20 and males aged 20 and 80 years (MDRD equation). For a male with a serum creatinine = 240 micromol/L (2.7 mg/dL) altering the sex to female, or the age from 20 to 80 years, reduces the eGFR from 31 to 23 ml/min/1.73 m². The line for a male aged 80 is almost identical to that for a female aged 20 years

---

Patient 2.1: Biochemical 'Sex Change'

Mr Edwards was shocked to be told by his GP that he needed to go back to the kidney clinic and talk about possible dialysis because his kidney function had suddenly dropped from 25 to 18 (see Fig. 2.8).

Careful study of the laboratory report revealed the mistake:

```
Patient: 123456          John Edwards
Date of Birth 14/08/1948  Female
Sample B,13.0763622 (BLOOD)   Collected 16 Jun 2013 08:00
Received 16 Jun 2013 12:00
Urea & Electrolytes
     Sodium                141    mmol/L     (133 - 146)
     Potassium             5.0    mmol/L     (3.5 - 5.3)
     Urea         *        19.6   mmol/L     (2.5 - 7.8)
     Creatinine   *        235    µmol/L     (50 - 98)
     Estimated GFR  *      18     ml/min/1.73m²
```

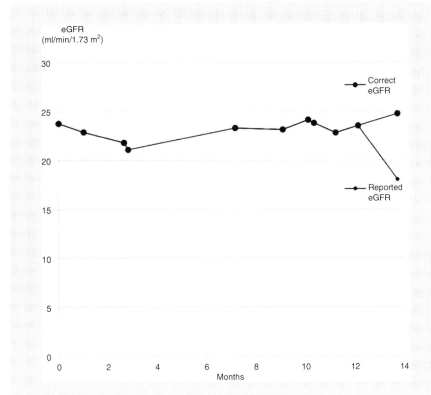

Fig. 2.8 Apparent drop in eGFR due to error on laboratory report

Patient 2.2: Biochemical 'Sex-Change'

Mrs Tracey Paul was delighted to be told at her routine diabetes clinic review that her kidney function had improved (see Fig. 2.9).

Unfortunately, the good news was an error; her kidney was declining after all. The error was picked up when a doctor questioned how serum creatinine and eGFR had both increased. Here is her laboratory report:

```
Patient: 234567          Tracey Paul
Date of Birth 02/07/1937      Male
Sample B, 13.0343712 (BLOOD)  Collected 15 Apr 2014 Received
15 Apr 2014 15:38
Urea & Electrolytes
     Sodium                139     mmol/L      (133 - 146)
     Potassium             4.9     mmol/L      (3.5 - 5.3)
     Urea          *       16.7    mmol/L      (2.5 - 7.8)
     Creatinine    *       144     µmol/L      (50 - 98)
     Estimated GFR *       41      ml/min/1.73m²
```

Previous results:

Date	Sodium	Potassium	Urea	Creatinine	eGFR
15.01.2014	141	5.0	14.8	126	37

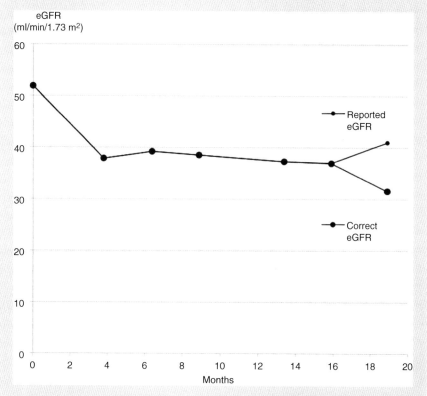

Fig. 2.9 Apparent rise in eGFR due to error on laboratory report

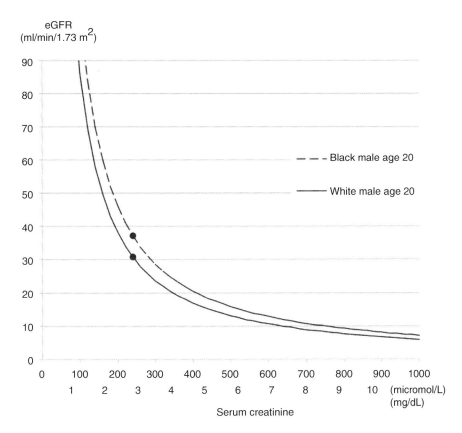

Fig. 2.10 eGFR (*filled circle*) calculated for white and black males aged 20 years (MDRD equation). For a man with a serum creatinine = 240 micromol/L (2.7 mg/dL), altering the race from white to black increases the eGFR by 21 %, from 31 to 37 ml/min/1.73 m²

Not All Changes in Serum Creatinine Are Caused by Changes in GFR

Changes in serum creatinine do not necessarily indicate changes in glomerular filtration. Three other factors affect the serum creatinine concentration: dietary creatinine, muscle mass and secretion of creatinine by the tubules.

Dietary Creatinine

Little creatinine is absorbed from meat in a usual diet. However, meat that has been boiled, such as in goulash, leads to a rise in creatinine that lasts 8 h. Dietary supplements, such as protein shakes and creatine, do not alter GFR [13] but there can be a transient increase in serum creatinine with excessive amounts. People who use these supplements do so to increase their muscle mass. Therefore it can be hard to work out whether a high serum creatinine level is due to the creatine supplements, a high muscle mass, reduced GFR, or a combination of all three.

In this situation, it is helpful to use an alternative maker of glomerular filtration to creatinine, namely cystatin C [14]. Cystatin C is a small protein comprising 120 amino acids that is produced by all nucleated cells, not just muscle. Its function is to inhibit enzymes that break down proteins, in particular extracellular cysteine proteases. It is freely filtered by glomeruli and then reabsorbed by the tubules; only small amounts are excreted in the urine.

Equations based upon cystatin C give a more accurate estimate of GFR when it is in the normal range and so are useful for distinguishing whether a raised serum creatinine is due to large muscle mass alone or a reduced GFR.

Patient 2.3: Big Muscles or Small Kidneys?
Emershan was a fit and healthy 33 year old black man. He had been a successful athlete, specialising in sprint distances. He had had his U&E's checked as part of a number of tests for chest pains, for which no cause was ever found. These were the results (Table 2.1).

Estimated GFR was 55 ml/min/1.73 m² (adjusted for black race)

His blood pressure was normal and urinalysis showed no blood or protein. Urinary albumin:creatinine ratio was 0.2 mg/mmol. A kidney ultrasound scan was normal.

He ate a normal diet with no creatine supplements.

He was anxious that he may have a kidney disease. To resolve the issue, serum cystatin C was measured. The result, 0.93 mg/L, gave an eGFR using the CKD-EPI Cystatin C (2012) equation of 95 ml/min/1.73 m². He was reassured.

Table 2.1 Emershan's blood results

Sodium	139 mmol/L	(133–146)		
Potassium	4.4 mmol/L	(3.5–5.3)		
Urea	4.3 mmol/L	(2.5–7.8)	BUN	12.0 mg/dL
Creatinine	130 micromol/L	(64–111)	Creatinine	1.47 mg/dL

Changes in Muscle Mass

Creatinine production is proportional to a patient's skeletal muscle mass. If a patient loses or gains a lot of muscle, the serum creatinine concentration will change independently of GFR. For example, patients who are seriously ill requiring care in an intensive therapy unit (ITU) can lose a substantial amount of body weight. As a result, their serum creatinine can be up to one-third lower after the illness. This reduces the apparent number of patients left with kidney damage on discharge from the ITU, and the severity of that damage as estimated from their serum creatinine [15].

Tubular Secretion of Creatinine

The equations used to estimate GFR take the tubular secretion of creatinine into account. However, problems arise when a patient is given a drug that blocks secretion of creatinine by the tubules. The most commonly used drug that does this is the antibiotic trimethoprim [16]. The anti-arrhythmic dronedarone has the same effect is some patients [17].

Treatment with these drugs will cause the eGFR to drop, even though the true GFR has not changed.

Patient 2.4: The Trimethoprim Effect

Rick, a longstanding kidney transplant patient receiving ciclosporin and prednisolone, was troubled by recurrent *Escherichia coli* urinary infections. These responded well to long-term treatment with alternating courses of trimethoprim and cephalexin. Each time Rick took trimethoprim the eGFR dropped and he was worried that his transplant was being damaged (Table 2.2).

The serum urea was the clue that the tubular effect of trimethoprim was causing a rise in creatinine. It did not rise with the serum creatinine, suggesting that the true GFR was unchanged.

Table 2.2 Sequential biochemical results in a kidney transplant patient receiving prophylactic antibiotics

Date	Urea (mmol/l)	Creatinine (micromol/L)	BUN (mg/dL)	Creatinine (mg/dL)	eGFR (ml/min/1.73 m^2)	Antibiotic
22 Oct 2013	13.3	168	37.3	1.90	40.2	TMP
05 Nov 2013	13.0	166	36.4	1.88	40.8	TMP
21 Jan 2014	12.6	136	35.3	1.54	51.5	Ceph
27 May 2014	11.7	167	32.8	1.89	40.4	TMP
26 Aug 2014	12.5	147	35.0	1.66	46.9	Ceph

TMP trimethoprim, *Ceph* cephalexin

Serum Urea and Creatinine – Different Measures of Kidney Function

Changes in serum urea can give useful additional information about what is happening to kidney function. Urea and creatinine are both filtered by the glomeruli but only urea can diffuse across cell membranes and be reabsorbed from the tubules.

The amount of urea reabsorbed is determined by the rate of flow of filtrate along the nephron. When the rate slows, more urea is reabsorbed and the rate of excretion falls (see Fig. 2.11).

How does this difference affect a patient's results? Consider two people: one with polycystic kidneys (ADPKD), the other with normal kidneys but low blood pressure due to prolonged diarrhoea. In the man with ADPKD, half of the nephrons have been affected by cysts and do not function – his GFR is half-normal. However, the rate of flow of filtrate in the functioning nephrons is normal and he produces a normal volume of urine per day.

In the man with low blood pressure, the nephrons are filtering at half the normal rate – his GFR is also half-normal. To compensate for the hypovolaemia, salt and water are reabsorbed from the tubules into the blood and the flow of filtrate along the nephrons is slow. Urine volume is reduced.

Because the glomerular filtration rate is halved, the concentration of creatinine is doubled in both patients. However, in the second patient, the slower flow of filtrate along the nephrons allows more urea to diffuse out of the tubules into the blood. As a result, the serum urea concentration is higher in the second patient than in the first.

Calculating the ratio of serum urea to serum creatinine shows this effect (Table 2.3).

A urea-to-creatinine ratio >100 (BUN-to-creatinine ratio >20) is often said to indicate dehydration but can occur in any situation in which the flow of filtrate along the nephrons is slowed. It is a marker of a pre-renal or, more precisely, pre-glomerular cause of kidney impairment.

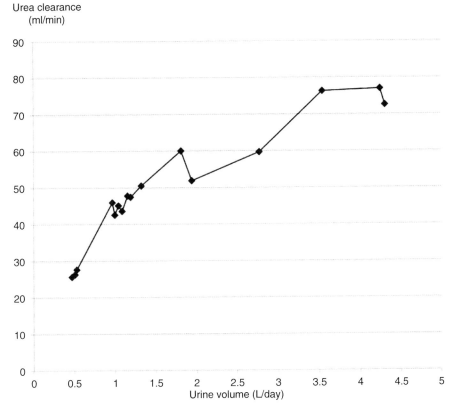

Fig. 2.11 Effect of urine volume on the rate of excretion of urea, calculated as the urea clearance. *Filled diagonal box* indicate measurements of serum creatinine (Redrawn from clearance values reported in [18]. Data are from samples taken from Harold Austin, published in 1921 [19])

Table 2.3 Calculation of the urea-to-creatinine ratio

	ADPKD	Low blood pressure
Urea (mmol/L)	10.2	33.5
BUN (mg/dL)	28.6	93.8
Creatinine (micromol/L)	160	160
Creatinine (mg/dL)	1.8	1.8
eGFR (ml/min/1.73 m²)	38.9	38.9
Urea-to-creatinine ratio	$10,200 \div 160 = \mathbf{63.8}$	$33,500 \div 160 = \mathbf{209.4}$
BUN-to-creatinine ratio	$28.6 \div 1.8 = \mathbf{15.9}$	$93.5 \div 1.8 = \mathbf{51.9}$

References

1. Shemesh O, Golbetz H, Kriss JP, Myers BD. Limitations of creatinine as a filtration marker in glomerulopathic patients. Kidney Int. 1985;28(5):830–8. http://www.nature.com/ki/journal/v28/n5/pdf/ki1985205a.pdf.
2. Levey AS, Bosch JP, Lewis JB, Greene T, Rogers N, Roth D. A more accurate method to estimate glomerular filtration rate from serum creatinine: a new prediction equation. Modification of Diet in Renal Disease Study Group. Ann Intern Med. 1999;130(6):461–70. PubMed: 10075613. http://annals.org/article.aspx?articleid=712617.
3. Schwartz GJ, Work DF. Measurement and estimation of GFR in children and adolescents. Clin J Am Soc Nephrol. 2009;4(11):1832–43. doi:10.2215/CJN.01640309. Published ahead of print October 9, 2009. http://cjasn.asnjournals.org/content/4/11/1832.full.
4. Schwartz GJ, Muñoz A, Schneider MF, Mak RH, Kaskel F, Warady BA, Furth SL. New equations to estimate GFR in children with CKD. J Am Soc Nephrol. 2009;20:629–37. doi:10.1681/ASN.2008030287. http://jasn.asnjournals.org/content/20/3/629.full.
5. Smith M, Moran P, Ward M, Davison J. Assessment of glomerular filtration rate during pregnancy using the MDRD formula. BJOG. 2008;115:109–12. http://onlinelibrary.wiley.com/doi/10.1111/j.1471-0528.2007.01529.x/full.
6. KDIGO 2012 Clinical Practice Guideline for the Evaluation and Management of Chronic Kidney Disease. www.kdigo.org/clinical_practice_guidelines/pdf/CKD/KDIGO_2012_CKD_GL.pdf; www.nice.org.uk/guidance/CG182/chapter/introduction.
7. Levey AS, Stevens LA, Schmid CH, Zhang YL, Castro 3rd AF, Feldman HI, Kusek JW, Eggers P, Van Lente F, Greene T, Coresh J, CKD-EPI (Chronic Kidney Disease Epidemiology Collaboration). A new equation to estimate glomerular filtration rate. Ann Intern Med. 2009;150(9):604–12. http://www.ncbi.nlm.nih.gov/pmc/articles/PMC2763564/.
8. Kilbride HS, Stevens PE, Eaglestone G, Knight S, Carter JL, Delaney MP, Farmer CK, Irving J, O'Riordan SE, Dalton RN, Lamb EJ. Accuracy of the MDRD (Modification of Diet in Renal Disease) study and CKD-EPI (CKD Epidemiology Collaboration) equations for estimation of GFR in the elderly. Am J Kidney Dis. 2013;61(1):57–66. doi:10.1053/j.ajkd.2012.06.016. Epub 2012 Aug 11. http://www.ajkd.org/article/S0272-6386(12)00941-9/abstract.
9. Xie D, Joffe MM, Brunelli SM, Beck G, Chertow GM, Fink JC, Greene T, Hsu C-Y, Kusek JW, Landis R, Lash J, Levey AS, O'Conner A, Ojo A, Rahman M, Townsend RR, Wang H, Feldman HI. A comparison of change in measured and estimated glomerular filtration rate in patients with nondiabetic kidney disease. Clin J Am Soc Nephrol. 2008;3(5):1332–8. http://www.ncbi.nlm.nih.gov/pmc/articles/PMC2518808/.
10. Padala S, Tighiouart H, Inker LA, Contreras G, Beck GJ, Lewis J, Steffes M, Rodby RA, Schmid CH, Levey AS. Accuracy of a GFR estimating equation over time in people with a wide range of kidney function. Am J Kidney Dis. 2012;60(2):217–24. http://www.ncbi.nlm.nih.gov/pmc/articles/PMC3399947/.
11. Franz KA, Reubl FC. Rate of functional deterioration in polycystic kidney disease. Kidney Int. 1983;23:526–9. http://www.nature.com/ki/journal/v23/n3/pdf/ki198351a.pdf.
12. Ama PF, Simoneau JA, Boulay MR, Serresse O, Thériault G, Bouchard C. Skeletal muscle characteristics in sedentary black and Caucasian males. J Appl Physiol (1985). 1986;61(5):1758–61. http://jap.physiology.org/content/61/5/1758.
13. Lugaresi R, Leme M, de Salles Painelli V, Murai IH, Roschel H, Sapienza MT, Herbert Lancha AH, Gualano B. Does long-term creatine supplementation impair kidney function in resistance-trained individuals consuming a high-protein diet? J Int Soc Sports Nutr. 2013;10:26. doi:10.1186/1550-2783-10-26. http://www.jissn.com/content/10/1/26.
14. Stevens LA, Coresh J, Schmid CH, Feldman HI, Froissart M, Kusek J, Rossert J, Van Lente F, Bruce RD, Zhang YL, Greene T, Levey AS. Estimating GFR using serum cystatin C alone and in combination with serum creatinine: a pooled analysis of 3418 individuals with CKD. Am J Kidney Dis. 2008;51(3):395–406. doi:10.1053/j.ajkd.2007.11.018. http://www.ncbi.nlm.nih.gov/pmc/articles/PMC2390827/.

15. Prowle JR, Kolic I, Purdell-Lewis J, Taylor R, Pearse RM, Kirwan CJ. Serum creatinine changes associated with critical illness and detection of persistent renal dysfunction after AKI. Clin J Am Soc Nephrol. 2014;9(6):1015–23. doi:10.2215/CJN.11141113. published ahead of print April 17, 2014, http://cjasn.asnjournals.org/content/9/6/1015.abstract.

16. Berg KJ, Gjellestad A, Nordby G, Rootwelt K, Djøseland O, Fauchald P, Mehl A, Narverud J, Talseth T. Renal effects of trimethoprim in ciclosporin- and azathioprine-treated kidney-allografted patients. Nephron. 1989;53(3):218–22. http://www.karger.com/Article/Abstract/185747.

17. Duncker D, Oswald H, Gardiwal A, Lüsebrink U, König T, Schreyer H, Klein G. Stable cystatin C serum levels confirm normal renal function in patients with dronedarone-associated increase in serum creatinine. J Cardiovasc Pharmacol Ther. 2013;18(2):109. http://cpt.sage-pub.com/content/18/2/109.abstract.

18. Van Slyke DD. The effect of urine volume on urea excretion. J Clin Invest. 1947;26:1159–67. http://www.ncbi.nlm.nih.gov/pmc/articles/PMC439461/pdf/jcinvest00386-0111.pdf.

19. Austin JH, Stillman E, Van Slyke DD. Factors governing the excretion rate of urea. J Biol Chem. 1921;46:91–112. http://www.jbc.org/content/46/1/91.full.pdf.

Chapter 3
Plot All the Dots

Graphs Reveal the Progression of Kidney Disease

Abstract In this chapter we explain:

- The importance of plotting a complete eGFR graph
- How to analyse variation in eGFR over time
- How serum creatinine changes in acute kidney injury
- How acute and chronic kidney disease are interlinked

Good doctors are skilled at taking a patient's history. As Sir William Osler[1] famously said: "Listen to your patient, he is telling you the diagnosis".

But patients with kidney disease often have no symptoms, so Osler's advice can be modified to: "Look at your patient's eGFR graph, it is telling you the kidney history".

In other words:

Plot all
the dots!

---

[1] William Osler (1849–1919), a Canadian physician, was one of the four founding professors of Johns Hopkins Hospital in Baltimore, Maryland, United States. Osler created the first speciality training program for physicians and was the first to provide bedside clinical training. He has been described as the "Father of Modern Medicine".

© Springer International Publishing Switzerland 2016
H. Rayner et al., *Understanding Kidney Diseases*,
DOI 10.1007/978-3-319-23458-8_3

Viewing the results as a column of figures is not enough; your brain cannot adjust for the different time intervals between the results to see the trends. Also, there may be so many results that you cannot view them all at once. Simply drawing a graph overcomes all these problems [1].

The graph helps both clinicians and patients to make sense of what is happening. And with this understanding, the patient is more likely to be motivated to modify their lifestyle or adhere to a drug treatment.

The more complete the dataset the better. It may require some detective work and telephone calls to pathology laboratories to track down all the old results (Patient 3.1). You may need to convert previous serum creatinine results into estimated GFR values, as explained in Chap. 2. These GFR estimates may be less accurate than those provided by the laboratory as they may use uncorrected serum creatinine values. However, they give valuable information about long-term trends in kidney function.

Patient 3.1: Hunting Out the History

Arthur, a 70 year old man with diabetes, was referred by his GP for advice about how to improve the control of his blood pressure and glucose. This is a table of his eGFR results for the previous 2½ years (Table 3.1).

The variation in the time intervals between the results makes it hard to interpret the table of numbers. A graph of the results resolves this problem (Fig. 3.1).

The variation between these results makes it difficult to estimate the rate of decline in GFR. Further searching of the laboratory database uncovered some older results that had been stored using a different patient identification number. The pathology database had not automatically merged these with the more recent records. When this was done manually, the trend over 10 years was revealed (Fig. 3.2).

Table 3.1 Sequential eGFR results over 2½ years

	eGFR
18 Apr 2011	51.3
07 Nov 2011	47.8
10 Feb 2012	52.0
23 Jul 2012	37.9
20 Aug 2012	51.5
10 Oct 2012	56.4
29 Jul 2013	44.5
30 Oct 2013	46.1

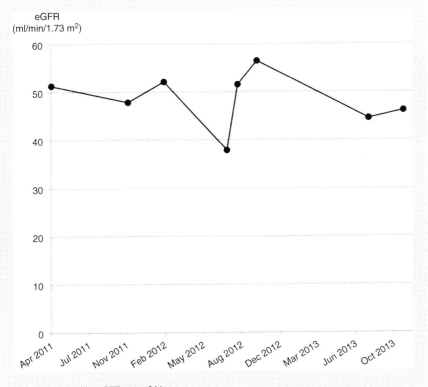

Fig. 3.1 Trend in eGFR over 2½ years

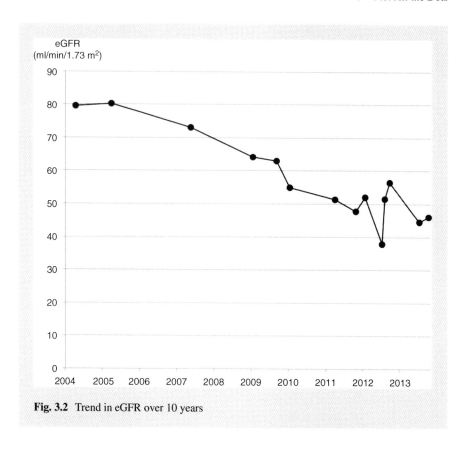

Fig. 3.2 Trend in eGFR over 10 years

Once you have tracked down all the eGFR results and plotted a complete graph, the next step is to interpret it correctly.

Analysing Variation in eGFR

If you took blood from the same person every day for 1 week, the seven serum creatinine results would not all be the same. They would vary above and below an average value. This is caused by variation in the person's true GFR from day to day combined with variation in the laboratory assay.

The minimum difference between two measurements that is statistically significant is called the Reference Change Value (RCV). The RCV is calculated by combining the biological and analytical variation of the substance being analysed. The RCV for eGFR at an eGFR of 60 is 10 ml/min/1.73 m². At an eGFR of 30 it is 6 ml/min/1.73 m² [2].

These figures suggest that eGFR is an insensitive way of measuring changes in kidney function. However, the RCV is a statistical comparison of only two values. Patients with kidney disease usually have many more than two readings to compare. Comparing multiple values averages out the analytical variation, making the trend in the eGFR a reliable and sensitive way to detect change in kidney function [3].

When we analyse a series of eGFR values we want to know whether the latest result is significantly different from the previous ones. Does it indicate a real change in the patient's health or is it within the expected range of variation of their known condition. In other words, is the patient's kidney function stable?

'Stable' is used as a mathematical term. It means that both the mean eGFR and the range of variation either side of the mean are constant over time. If the eGFR is stable, the mean is stationary and there are no non-random signals.

The comparative statistics used in the RCV are not helpful for analyzing sequential or time-series data. We need to use different statistical tests.

To test whether the output of a process is stable, sequential data are plotted on a chart called a run chart. The eGFR graph is a type of run chart. If we have sufficient data points, usually more than 20, the range of expected variation can be estimated using Statistical Process Control (SPC).

To perform an SPC analysis, upper and lower control limits, sometimes called natural process limits, are drawn on the chart. They indicate the range beyond which the process output, in this case the eGFR, is statistically unlikely to occur by chance, i.e. about 3 in a 1000. If the variation remains within the control limits, the process is said to be stable. If data points deviate outside the limits or meet statistical tests for a non-random pattern, the process is unstable and a 'special cause' is indicated [4].

An SPC chart can sometimes be helpful for analysing a series of eGFR results.

Patient 3.2: Using an SPC Chart to Analyse Variation in eGFR

Marjorie was aged 82 and had CKD stage 4 due to diabetes and hypertension. Her eGFR was stable over 5 years. She then presented to hospital with cellulitis of her leg and hypotension. She was treated with antibiotics and allowed home.

Reviewing her eGFR results, the value on presentation was below the lower control limit (LCL) on a SPC chart drawn using all her previous results (BaseLine©, www.SAASoft.com) (Fig. 3.3). This was a warning that the sepsis was affecting her kidneys.

Six weeks later she returned to hospital more unwell. Her eGFR had dropped to 5 ml/min/1.73 m^2. The clinical significance of the value taken previously was now clear (Fig. 3.4).

With intensive treatment over the following month her eGFR returned to its previous mean baseline.

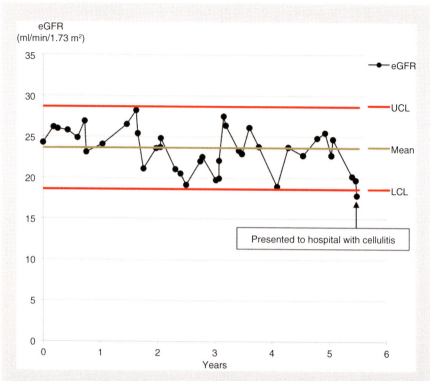

Fig. 3.3 Statistical Process Control chart of eGFR values over 5 years. When the patient presented to hospital with cellulitis, the eGFR was below the lower control limit. This indicates that the deviation was significantly greater than expected from the previous normal variation for the patient. *UCL* upper control limit, *LCL* lower control limit

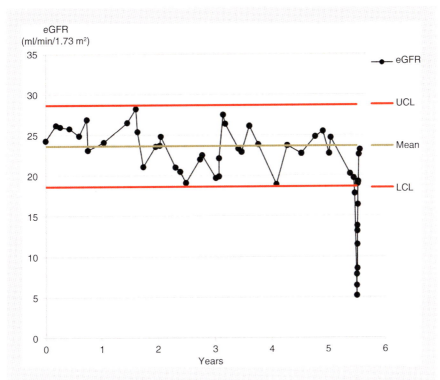

Fig. 3.4 Statistical Process Control chart showing acute kidney injury with recovery to previous baseline. *UCL* upper control limit, *LCL* lower control limit

Unfortunately, an SPC approach to analysing eGFR results is usually not possible for a number of reasons. Firstly, measurements of eGFR may be too infrequent or few in number to provide a reliable baseline. Secondly, kidney function is more likely to be measured when a patient is unwell and so the results may not be representative of the healthy baseline. And finally, the underlying GFR is often declining over time and so the mean is unstable. An SPC chart cannot be used to interpret variation about an unstable mean.

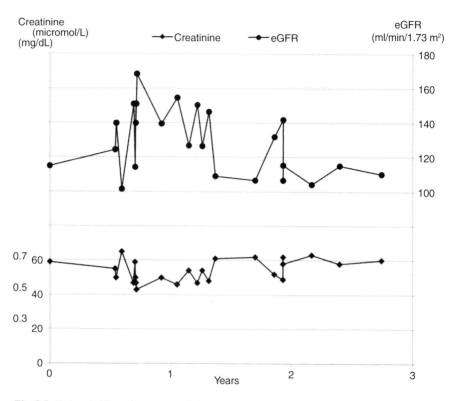

Fig. 3.5 Patient 1: Normal serum creatinine – wide variation in eGFR

Interpreting Variation in an eGFR Graph

Variation in eGFR is greatest at low levels of serum creatinine because of the inverse relationship between creatinine and eGFR. Figures 3.5 and 3.6 are charts from two kidney transplant patients. The first patient (Fig. 3.5) has good transplant function and normal serum creatinine; the average eGFR is high and the variation is wide. The second patient (Fig. 3.6) has poor function and high serum creatinine; the average eGFR is low and the variation is narrow.

The range of variation in eGFR also depends upon the underlying kidney disease. Patients with wide variation in GFR may be having multiple episodes of 'micro' acute kidney injury. This pattern is associated with a greater risk of decline in eGFR over the long term and an increased risk of mortality [5].

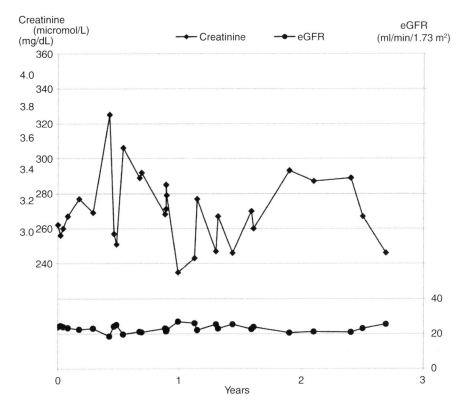

Fig. 3.6 Patient 2: High serum creatinine – narrow variation in eGFR

Patient 3.3: Wide Variation in eGFR Predicts a Poor Outcome
Natasha had type 1 diabetes. Her blood glucose control had been very poor despite a multiple daily dose regimen, so she used an insulin pump. To make matters worse, she had Addison's disease and suffered from recurrent urinary infections. Infections caused her to have Addisonian crises with hypotension and acute kidney injury. Her eGFR varied widely for a number of years and then showed a declining trend (Fig. 3.7). As the eGFR fell, the variation around the trendline narrowed.

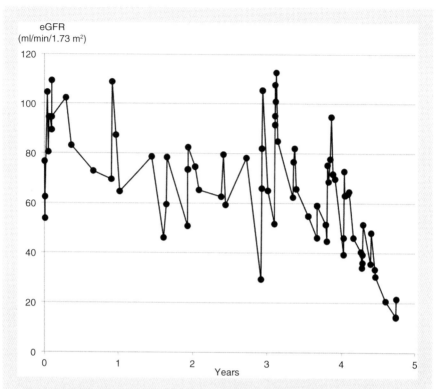

Fig. 3.7 Variation in eGFR in a patient with diabetes, urinary infections and Addison's disease. Wide variation over 4 years preceded a rapid decline in eGFR

Clinical judgement and experience are needed to interpret eGFR graphs; it is a skill that requires practice. The more you use graphs of eGFR and other clinical measurements, the more skilled you will become at seeing links – sometimes unexpected ones – between changes in data and clinical events. You can become familiar with common patterns in graphs by studying the examples throughout this book, such as Patient 3.4.

Patient 3.4: Interpreting a More Complex eGFR Graph
Mr Fish was 76 years old. He had diabetes and so had regular checks of his kidney function. Here is his eGFR graph (Fig. 3.8).

The graph can be divided into four periods (Fig. 3.9).

In the first period, the eGFR values are between 70 and 50 ml/min/1.73 m^2 and the trend is slowly downwards due to his advancing age and diabetic nephrosclerosis.

In the second period, the trend turns abruptly downwards. Mr Fish was
unaware that his poor urinary stream and occasional incontinence were due
to chronic urinary retention. It was only after a number of eGFR measurements showing worsening function that he was referred to a nephrologist,
who palpated his grossly distended bladder.

At the start of the third period, a urinary catheter was inserted. This led to a
rapid initial improvement in eGFR followed by a slower increase.

In the fourth period, the eGFR varies above and below a stable mean eGFR of
35 ml/min/1.73 m², indicating residual non-progressive kidney damage.

This example comes from a time when eGFR was not routinely reported.
One wonders how much of Mr Fish's kidney function could have been saved
if the decline in his eGFR during period 2 had been noticed and acted upon
sooner.

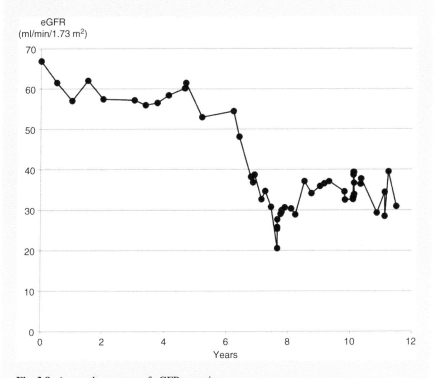

Fig. 3.8 A complex pattern of eGFR over time

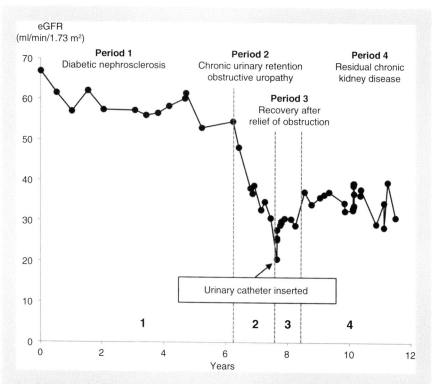

Fig. 3.9 Interpretation of the eGFR graph as a sequence of four periods with different pathological processes

Acute Kidney Injury – Equilibrating Creatinine

The serum creatinine concentration is only a reliable maker of kidney function when it is in a steady state. Production and excretion of creatinine need to be in equilibrium. In acute kidney disease things are not in equilibrium; the creatinine concentration increases as the GFR decreases and vice versa.

The time it takes to reach equilibrium is demonstrated by the surgical removal of a kidney for carcinoma. When the renal artery is clamped off there is an immediate step down in the patient's total GFR due to the loss of the function of one kidney. At the moment the artery is clamped the serum creatinine is unchanged and over the subsequent 24 h it progressively increases until a new equilibrium is reached (Fig. 3.10).

During this 24 h period, the creatinine concentration lags behind the true GFR. Twenty four hours after the step down in GFR the creatinine concentration has reached a new equilibrium.

Serum creatinine
(micromol/L)

Serum creatinine
(mg/dL)

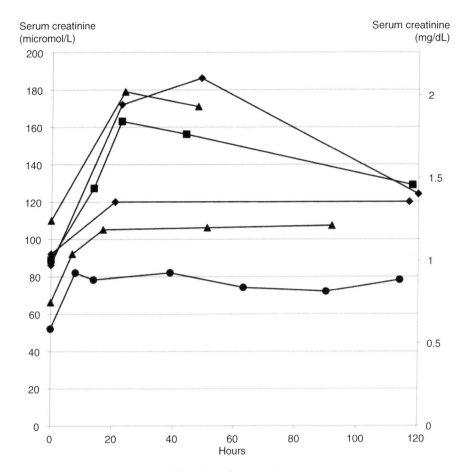

Fig. 3.10 Serum creatinine values following unilateral nephrectomy in six patients

The size of the increase depends upon the function that the kidney had before it was removed. In some patients the creatinine concentration falls over the following days as their remaining kidney's GFR increases (Fig. 3.10). The fall parallels direct measurements of GFR in an experimental rat model, which show a small increase in GFR beginning 24 h after unilateral nephrectomy [6].

The magnitude of the percentage rise in serum creatinine and the peak value reached are used to categorise acute kidney injury into three stages of severity, defined by their associated mortality risk (Table 3.2) [7].

The initial diagnosis or detection of acute kidney injury is based upon a patient meeting any of the criteria for Stage 1. Staging is carried out retrospectively when the episode is complete. Patients are classified according to the highest possible stage where the criterion is met, either by creatinine rise or by urine output.

Table 3.2 Detection and staging of acute kidney injury in adults according to Kidney Disease Improving Global Outcomes (KDIGO)

Stage	Creatinine	Urine volume
1	Rise of ≥26 mmol/l[a] or 0.3 mg/dl within 48 h Or 50–99 % Cr rise from baseline within 7 days[b] (1.50–1.99×baseline)	<0.5 ml/kg/h for more than 6 h
2	100–199 % Cr rise from baseline within 7 days[b] (2.00–2.99×baseline)	<0.5 ml/kg/h for more than 12 h
3	≥200 % Cr rise from baseline within 7 days[b] (≥3×baseline) Or (current) Cr >354 mmol/l (4.0 mg/dL) with either: rise of ≥26 mmol/l[a] or 0.3 mg/dl within 48 h or ≥50 % Cr rise from baseline within 7 days[b] Or any requirement for renal replacement therapy	<0.3 ml/kg/h for 24 h Or anuria for 12 h

Abbreviations: *Cr* creatinine
[a]SI units rounded down to the nearest integer
[b]Where the rise is known (based on a prior blood test) or presumed (based on the patient history) to have occurred within 7 days

Illness that is severe enough to cause acute kidney injury, such as sepsis, can also reduce the production of creatinine by skeletal muscle so the change in serum creatinine may underestimate the drop in GFR [8].

Dealing with Missing Data

Acute kidney injury is often unexpected and the patient may not have had their serum creatinine measured shortly before the illness. This can make it difficult to decide whether someone has AKI and to gauge its severity. One cannot assume the creatinine was previously in the normal range. Indeed patients with AKI are more likely to have underlying chronic kidney disease.

Many ways have been explored to overcome this difficulty [7]. One option is to take an average of previous readings and use that number as the baseline to calculate the AKI stage. This is simple but potentially misleading. An average does not take into account the sequence of the values being averaged.

Figures 3.11 and 3.12 contain the same values of eGFR. The average of the first five results is shown as a horizontal dashed line. In the first chart (Fig. 3.11) the latest result has dropped compared to the average baseline. Using this definition the patient has suffered either acute kidney injury (defined as a decline occurring over ≤7 days) or acute kidney disease (defined as a decline occurring over 7–90 days).

In the second chart (Fig. 3.12), the average is the same but the baseline results show a declining trend. The latest result is in line with this trend. The patient has progressive chronic kidney disease rather than acute kidney injury or disease.

There is no substitute for plotting all the dots to see what is really going on. If even that does not tell the story, it is best to play safe and assume that the decline is due to acute kidney injury and to look for a possible cause.

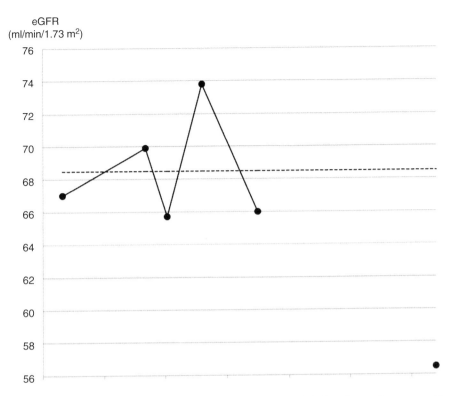

Fig. 3.11 Acute kidney injury – the latest eGFR measurement is below the previous range of variation. The average of the first five results is shown as a *horizontal dashed line*

Acute-On-Chronic Kidney Disease – Time in Two Dimensions

Kidney diseases have traditionally been divided into acute and chronic. This may be convenient for explaining different pathological processes but in practice the distinction is not so clear-cut.

There is a tendency, particularly in the hospital setting, to focus on the acute time dimension and overlook the chronic. If you plot the whole eGFR graph, rather than reading only the last few results, you will see both time dimensions (Fig. 3.13).

Acute and chronic kidney diseases are interlinked:

- Patients are more likely to suffer acute kidney injury if they have chronic kidney disease
- Patients who suffer acute kidney injury are commonly left with some chronic kidney disease and are more likely to develop high blood pressure
- Patients who suffer multiple episodes of acute kidney injury are more likely to progress to end-stage kidney failure and to die [9]

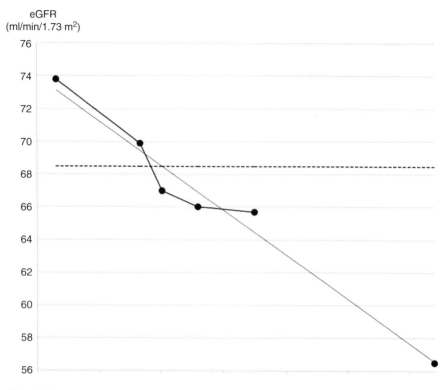

Fig. 3.12 Progressive chronic kidney disease – the latest eGFR measurement is on the linear trendline projected from the previous values. The average of the first five results is shown as a *horizontal dashed line*

Figure 3.14 shows the eGFR graph from a 58-year-old female smoker with long-standing hypertension. She suffered acute kidney injury at the time of her first myocardial infarction and was left with chronic kidney disease Stage G3. Two years later she suffered a second myocardial infarction that led to further acute and chronic loss of kidney function. She died suddenly at home 18 months later, presumably from another cardiac event.

The pathological link between AKI and CKD appears to be the failure of tubules damaged in the episode of acute injury to regenerate fully. The tubular cells do not differentiate into normal tubules and instead stimulate fibrosis in the interstitium. After a single injury the fibrotic scar remains limited to the region of the damaged tubules. However, repeated acute injury on top of chronic damage stimulates progressive spreading fibrosis and glomerular damage [10].

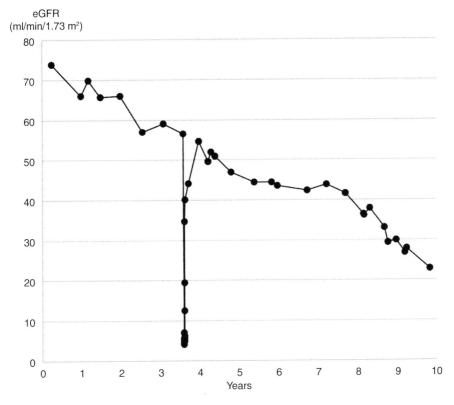

Fig. 3.13 eGFR graph from a man with diabetes who suffered an episode of severe gastroenteritis. Kidney function related to diabetic nephropathy changed over 10 years; kidney function related to gastroenteritis changed over 10 days

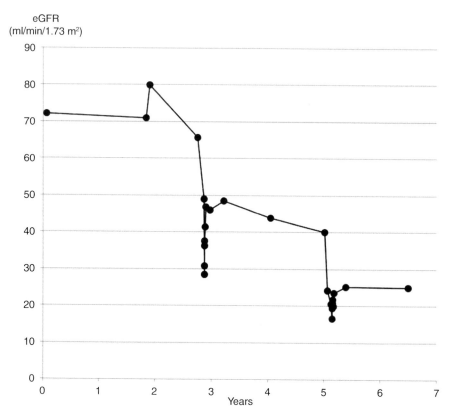

Fig. 3.14 Two episodes of AKI leading to CKD

References

1. Morgan DB, Will EJ. Selection, presentation, and interpretation of biochemical data in renal failure. Kidney Int. 1983;24:438–45. http://www.nature.com/ki/journal/v24/n4/abs/ki1983180a.html.
2. Badrick T, Turner P. The uncertainty of the eGFR. Indian J Clin Biochem. 2013;28(3):242–7. http://link.springer.com/article/10.1007%2Fs12291-012-0280-1.
3. Padala S, Tighiouart H, Inker LA, Contreras G, Beck GJ, Lewis J, Steffes M, Rodby RA, Schmid CH, Levey AS. Accuracy of a GFR estimating equation over time in people with a wide range of kidney function. Am J Kidney Dis. 2012;60(2):217–24. http://www.ncbi.nlm.nih.gov/pmc/articles/PMC3399947/.
4. Carey RG. Improving healthcare with control charts: basic and advanced SPC methods and case studies. Milwaukee: ASQ Quality Press; 2003. ISBN 0-87389-562-2.
5. Turin TC, Coresh J, Tonelli M, Stevens PE, de Jong PE, Farmer CKT, Matsushita K, Hemmelgarn BR. Change in the estimated glomerular filtration rate over time and risk of all-cause mortality. Kidney Int. 2013;83:684–91. doi:10.1038/ki.2012.443. http://www.nature.com/ki/journal/v83/n4/full/ki2012443a.html.

6. Chamberlain RM, Shirley DG. Time course of the renal functional response to partial nephrectomy: measurements in conscious rats. Exp Physiol. 2007;92:251–62. http://onlinelibrary.wiley.com/doi/10.1113/expphysiol.2006.034751/full.

7. Thomas ME, Blaine C, Dawnay A, Devonald MAJ, Ftouh S, Laing C, Latchem S, Lewington A, Milford DV, Ostermann M. The definition of acute kidney injury and its use in practice. Kidney Int. 2014. doi:10.1038/ki.2014.328. http://www.nature.com/ki/journal/v87/n1/full/ki2014328a.html.

8. Doi K, Yuen PST, Eisner C, Hu X, Leelahavanichkul A, Schnermann J, Star RA. Reduced production of creatinine limits its use as marker of kidney injury in sepsis. J Am Soc Nephrol. 2009;20:1217–21. doi:10.1681/ASN.2008060617. http://jasn.asnjournals.org/content/20/6/1217.abstract.

9. Horne KL, Packington R, Monaghan J, Reilly T, McIntyre CW, Selby NM. The effects of acute kidney injury on long-term renal function and proteinuria in a general hospitalised population. Nephron Clin Pract. 2014;128:192–200. doi:10.1159/000368243. http://www.karger.com/Article/Abstract/368243.

10. Venkatachalam MA, Weinberg JM, Kriz W, Bidani AK. Failed tubule recovery, AKI-CKD transition, and kidney disease progression. J Am Soc Nephrol. ASN.2015010006; doi:10.1681/ASN.2015010006. http://jasn.asnjournals.org/content/early/2015/03/25/ASN.2015010006.abstract.

Chapter 4
How Are You Feeling?

The Symptoms of Uraemia

Abstract In this chapter we explain:

- How symptoms change as kidney function declines
- How uraemia affects the nervous system

Stages of CKD

As the GFR declines, symptoms and signs of kidney failure become more common and more severe (see Fig. 4.1). To reflect that, CKD is graded into five stages by eGFR: G1–G5.

Patients with eGFR >60 need to have other evidence of kidney disease, such as proteinuria or a structural abnormality, to qualify as having Stage G1 (eGFR >90) or Stage G2 (eGFR 60–89). Stage G3 is divided into G3a (eGFR 45–60 ml/min/1.73 m^2) and G3b (eGFR 30–45). Stage G4 is eGFR 15–29 ml/min/1.73 m^2 and G5 is eGFR <15 ml/min/1.73 m^2.

The definition of CKD requires two reduced eGFR readings at least 3 months apart to confirm that the disease is chronic and implications for health to justify the term 'disease'. The full classification of someone with CKD requires the underlying cause, the eGFR and the level of albuminuria (see Sect. "Proteinuria" in page 143) [1].

Kidney failure does not make you feel very ill until it is advanced, so taking a history from a patient with kidney disease is little help in judging kidney function. The severity of symptoms experienced at a given level of eGFR varies considerably between individuals, some people remaining asymptomatic despite very low function.

The duration of symptoms is not a reliable guide to how quickly kidney failure has developed. Patients with chronic kidney disease may present acutely after a long period of symptomless disease (see Patient 4.1).

© Springer International Publishing Switzerland 2016
H. Rayner et al., *Understanding Kidney Diseases*,
DOI 10.1007/978-3-319-23458-8_4

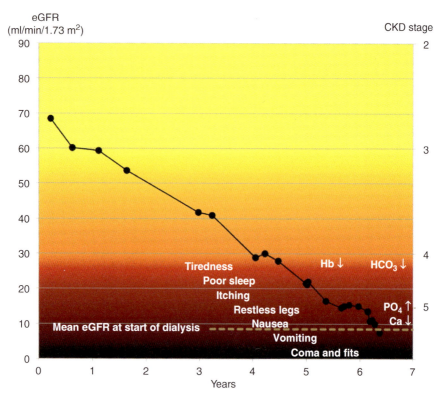

Fig. 4.1 The common symptoms experienced by patients at different stages of chronic kidney disease

Uraemia and the Nervous System

As GFR falls below 45 the commonest symptom is fatigue, defined as extreme and persistent tiredness, weakness or exhaustion – either mental, physical or both [2]. Patients whose GFR declines very slowly and are otherwise well may adjust their lifestyle and expectations to their gradually increasing fatigue.

As GFR declines below 20, symptoms such as insomnia, restless legs and itching (uraemic pruritus) increase.

Restless legs syndrome is a curious unpleasant symptom that patients characteristically find hard to describe. They refer to throbbing, pulling or creeping sensations inside their legs and have an uncontrollable urge to move them. The symptoms are worse when relaxing and are often worst at night. Moving the legs temporarily eases the feeling.

Itching is a major debilitating symptom for some patients with CKD stage G5, both before and after starting dialysis. Its constant presence, especially at night, leads to exhaustion and depression (Patient 4.1). Severe itching is even associated with increased mortality [3].

Patient 4.1: Severe Uraemic Pruritus

Vanessa had been on dialysis for 12 years. Over recent months, she had suffered from severe itching that stopped her getting to sleep and disrupted her family life. The itching on her back was so bad that she used an old belt to scratch herself, making her skin bleed.

She describes her symptoms in a video interview at vimeo.com/49458473 (Fig. 4.2).

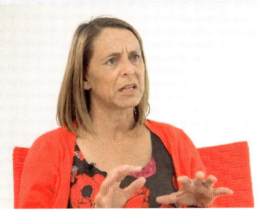

Fig. 4.2 Screenshot of video at http://vimeo. com/49458473

Itching due to kidney failure - A patient's experience

The itching may be associated with dry skin but there is usually no rash. Constant scratching causes bleeding and scarring (see Figs. 4.3 and 4.4).

The pathophysiology of these symptoms is not fully understood. As they often occur together, it is likely they are mediated by neuronal 'over activity' possibly due to the effects of uraemia on the nervous system [4].

Treatment of severe insomnia, restless legs and itching requires careful use of drugs that modify neurotransmission. Gabapentin and pregabalin can be particularly helpful for all these symptoms [5, 6]. The effect of gabapentin on itching is often dramatic, a single tablet switching off the symptom (Patient 4.1 continued). This supports the theory that itch is caused by excessive activity of the nerve fibres that transmit the sensation [7].

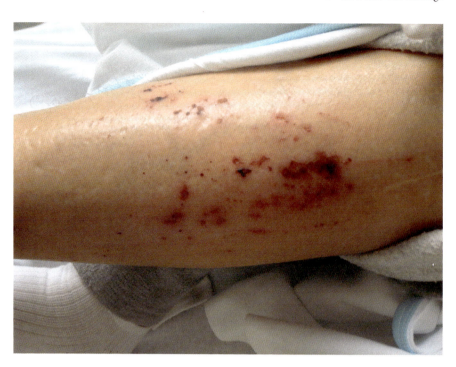

Fig. 4.3 Bleeding caused by scratching due to uraemic pruritus (Photograph courtesy of Prof. Dr. med. Thomas Mettang)

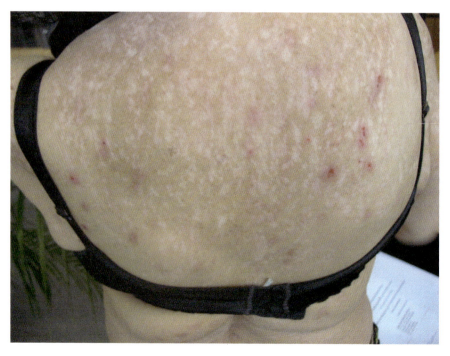

Fig 4.4 Scratch marks and scarring caused by persistent scratching due to uraemic pruritus (Photograph courtesy of Prof. Dr. med. Thomas Mettang)

Patient 4.1 continued: Treatment of Uraemic Pruritus with Gabapentin
Vanessa was offered treatment with gabapentin. After the first tablet the itching stopped almost completely.

  She describes the effect of the treatment and the impact this had on her life in a video interview at vimeo.com/49455976 (Fig. 4.5).

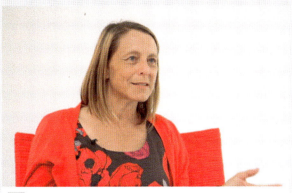

Fig. 4.5 Screenshot of video at http://vimeo.com/49455976

Gabapentin treatment for itching - A patient's experience

As GFR declines below 15, the fatigue becomes more marked and people readily fall asleep during the day. They may lose their appetite and feel sick, particularly if they have a diet high in protein. The sickness is typically worse in the mornings and there may be a bad taste in the mouth. The loss of appetite can lead to weight loss and eventually malnutrition.

When GFR reaches very low levels, patients suffer recurrent vomiting and a uraemic smell may be detected on their breath. A pericardial rub may be heard due to uraemic pericarditis.

People with underlying cerebral impairment such as dementia become more drowsy and confused. Peripheral neuropathy can cause weakness, numbness and ataxia from loss of proprioception. Without dialysis, patients may suffer seizures, delirium and eventually lapse into a coma prior to death.

These neurological complications can be exacerbated by dialysis. Rapid changes in the biochemistry of the blood cause disequilibrium across the blood-brain barrier. The reduction in the osmotic pressure in the blood causes fluid to cross the blood-brain barrier into the brain leading to cerebral oedema.

In the UK, the mean eGFR when people start dialysis is 8.5 ml/min/1.73 m^2, although some feel well despite having an eGFR below this. An extreme example (Patient 4.2) was a man who only presented to hospital when his eGFR reached 1.4 ml/min/1.73 m^2!

Patient 4.2: Extreme Results

Amar, a 20-year-old computer science student, had become increasing unwell over the previous 2 months with loss of appetite, weight loss, weakness, pain in the legs and tremors. His walking had become increasingly unsteady. He had continued his studies until this recent illness.

On admission, his blood pressure was 150/87, a loud pericardial rub was heard and he had bilateral leg oedema. An echocardiogram showed severe left ventricular hypertrophy with systolic and diastolic dysfunction.

In his legs there were signs of peripheral neuropathy with numbness, an ataxic gait and bilateral foot drop. Subsequent neurophysiology tests showed severe axonal sensory and motor polyneuropathy.

Both kidneys were grossly atrophic and difficult to see on an ultrasound scan. The right measured 5.5 cm and the left 5 cm in length. The renal cortices were extremely thin.

Here are his blood results (Table 4.1).

He was started on haemodialysis, initially via a femoral vein haemodialysis catheter. His first session was for 3 h at a relatively slow blood pump speed of 150 ml/min. This was to reduce the risk of disequilibrium syndrome from the first dialysis.

The dose of dialysis that is delivered can be estimated from the percentage by which urea is reduced during the treatment, the Urea Reduction Ratio (URR):

$$URR = \frac{\text{Predialysis urea concentration} - \text{Postdialysis urea concentration}}{\text{Predialysis urea concentration.}}$$

The goal for a regular dialysis treatment is >65 %. His first treatment achieved only 40.8 %. Despite these precautions, he suffered a generalised tonic-clonic seizure near the end of dialysis.

He was severely anaemic, haemoglobin = 49 g/L (4.9 g/dL), so was given a blood transfusion and started on erythropoietin. The pain from the peripheral neuropathy was treated with amitriptyline and gabapentin and he wore foot drop supports.

With daily dialysis for the first 2 weeks then three times a week he steadily improved. After 6 months he could walk without assistance. After 9 months an echocardiogram showed normal LV function.

A year after first presenting, he received a successful kidney transplant from his father.

Table 4.1 Blood results at the time Amar presented to hospital

		Normal range	Non-SI units
Sodium	125 mmol/L	133–146	125 mEq/L
Potassium	5.8 mmol/L	3.5–5.3	5.8 mEq/L
Urea	104.9 mmol/L	2.5–7.8	BUN 294 mg/dL
Creatinine	3378 micromol/L	64–111	38.2 mg/dL
eGFR	1.4 ml/min/1.73 m^2		
Bicarbonate	7.2 mmol/L	22.0–29.0	Total CO_2 7.2 mEq/L
Albumin	33 g/L	35–50	3.3 g/dL
Calcium (corrected for serum albumin)	1.44 mmol/L	2.20–2.60	5.8 mg/dL
Phosphate	5.17 mmol/L	0.80–1.50	Phosphorus 16.0 mg/dL
Alkaline phosphatase	63 IU/L	30–130	

References

1. Kidney Disease: Improving Global Outcomes (KDIGO) CKD Work Group. KDIGO 2012 clinical practice guideline for the evaluation and management of chronic kidney disease. Kidney Int Suppl. 2013;3:1–150. http://kdigo.org/home/guidelines/ckd-evaluation-management/.
2. Artom M, Moss-Morris R, Caskey F, Chilcot J. Fatigue in advanced kidney disease. Kidney Int. 2014;86:497–505. doi:10.1038/ki.2014.86. http://www.nature.com/ki/journal/v86/n3/full/ki201486a.html.
3. Pisoni RL, Wikstrom B, Elder SJ, et al. Pruritus in haemodialysis patients: international result from the Dialysis Outcomes and Practice Patterns Study (DOPPS). Nephrol Dial Transplant. 2006;21:3495–505. http://ndt.oxfordjournals.org/content/21/12/3495.full.
4. Mettang T, Kremer AE. Uremic pruritus. Kidney Int. 2015;87:685–91. doi:10.1038/ki.2013.454. http://www.nature.com/ki/journal/v87/n4/full/ki2013454a.html.
5. Gunal AI, Ozalp G, Yoldas TK, Gunal SY, Kirciman E, Celiker H. Gabapentin therapy for pruritus in haemodialysis patients: a randomized, placebo-controlled, double-blind trial. Nephrol Dial Transplant. 2004;19:3137–9. http://ndt.oxfordjournals.org/content/19/12/3137.full.pdf.
6. Yue J, Jiao S, Xiao Y, Ren W, Zhao T, Meng J. Comparison of pregabalin with ondansetron in treatment of uraemic pruritus in dialysis patients: a prospective, randomized, double-blind study. Int Urol Nephrol. 2014. doi:10.1007/s11255-014-0795-x. http://download.springer.com/static/pdf/823/art%253A10.1007%252Fs11255-014-0795-x.pdf?auth66=1425491040_c2475cbe1d116e09fa6998febcb2b056&ext=.pdf.
7. Rayner H, Baharani J, Smith S, Suresh V, Dasgupta I. Uraemic pruritus: relief of itching by gabapentin and pregabalin. Nephron Clin Pract. 2013;122(3–4):75–9. doi:10.1159/000349943. https://www.karger.com/Article/FullText/349943.

Chapter 5
Do You Have Any Long-Term Health Conditions?

Kidney Involvement in Multisystem Diseases

Abstract In this chapter we explain:

- How kidney disease develops in people with diabetes
- How vascular disease can affect the kidneys
- The effect of chronic infection and inflammation on the kidneys

Many diseases affect the kidneys as one part of a multisystem illness. They are included throughout the book and can be located using the index. Immune-mediated diseases are described in Chap. 14.

In this chapter we focus on the most common long term conditions that affect the kidneys – diabetes, atherosclerosis, and chronic infection and inflammation.

Diabetes Mellitus

The prevalence of diabetes worldwide is growing at an alarming rate. The rise has been almost exponential in the UK and the prevalence is likely to get worse as the obesity epidemic continues (Fig. 5.1).

Kidney involvement in diabetes is common; about 25 % of people with diabetes in England have proteinuria [1]. Although only 0.5 % has end-stage kidney failure, this percentage has more than doubled between 2004 and 2010. Diabetes is the commonest cause of chronic kidney disease; in some countries such as the US and Germany, up to half of patients with CKD attending nephrology clinics have diabetes.

The natural history of diabetic nephropathy typically progresses from microalbuminuria to macroalbuminuria and then to a decline in GFR. GFR increases in the initial stages of nephropathy and this hyperfiltration may accelerate damage to the glomeruli and increase albuminuria (see Fig. 5.2) [2].

© Springer International Publishing Switzerland 2016
H. Rayner et al., *Understanding Kidney Diseases*,
DOI 10.1007/978-3-319-23458-8_5

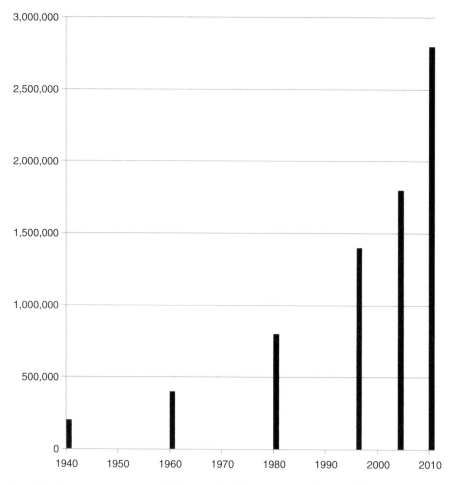

Fig. 5.1 The rising prevalence of diabetes in the UK over the last 70 years. Numbers of people affected (Data from various sources)

In more advanced disease, there is progressive sclerosis of glomeruli and the GFR declines, usually with a linear trend. The slope varies between patients, those with heavy proteinuria tending to decline more rapidly (see Fig. 5.3).

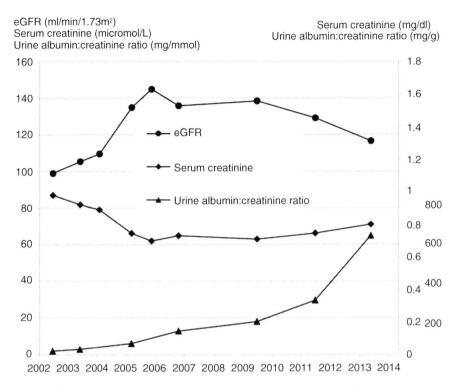

Fig. 5.2 The natural history of early diabetic nephropathy. There is steadily increasing albuminuria. GFR initially increases – 'hyperfiltration' – and then declines

Two factors increase the risk of someone with diabetes developing nephropathy – poor glucose control and high blood pressure. Achieving glucose control is particularly important in the first few years after diagnosis as this can leave a legacy of reduced risk in future years. Control needs to be achieved before albuminuria is established. In type 1 diabetes, the risk of reduced kidney function is halved by tight glucose control in the early years [3]. In type 2 diabetes, controlling blood glucose prevents the development of albuminuria but has no clear effect on the rate of decline in GFR [4]. Over-aggressive glucose control may be harmful. Intensive glucose treatment in people with kidney disease, even CKD stage 1, increases the risk of mortality by 30 % [5].

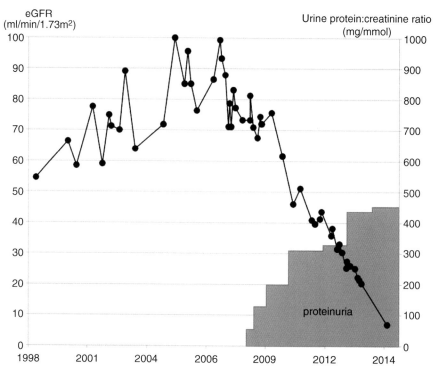

Fig. 5.3 The natural history of diabetic nephropathy showing hyperfiltration followed by heavy proteinuria and a decline in GFR to end stage kidney failure

Patient 5.1: Glucose Control Does Not Protect Against Loss of GFR
Andrea had type 1 diabetes since she was 8 years old and struggled for many years to control her blood glucose. In early 2013, aged 23 years, she attended a diabetes education course where she learned how to estimate her insulin needs and adjust the dose accordingly.

Her blood glucose control improved dramatically, as shown by the fall in glycated haemoglobin (HbA1c). Despite this, her GFR continued to decline (Fig. 5.4).

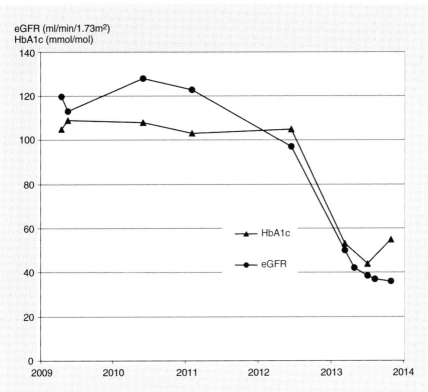

Fig. 5.4 Decline in GFR despite marked improvement in glucose control (HbA1c). 100 mmol/mol = 11.3 % DCCT. 50 mmol/mol = 6.7 % DCCT

With better treatment, especially using inhibitors of the renin-angiotensin-aldosterone system, outcomes in diabetic nephropathy have improved substantially in recent years [6]. Albuminuria can often be reduced, with microalbuminuria sometimes remitting completely [7]. Even patients with nephrotic-range proteinuria can benefit considerably from these drugs (see Patient 5.2).

Patient 5.2: The Effect of ACE Inhibition on Diabetic Nephropathy
Mr Archer had neglected his type 1 diabetes over many years and had failed to attend the diabetic clinic for long periods. He had developed peripheral and autonomic neuropathy, and suffered from postural hypotension and severe nocturnal and gustatory sweating.

He was persuaded to attend clinic by his partner who was increasingly concerned about his health. His blood pressure was high when seated (164/84) but low when he stood up (90/54). He had very swollen legs, nephrotic-range proteinuria (protein:creatinine ratio = 1148 mg/mmol) and hypoalbuminaemia (21 g/L); in other words he had the nephrotic syndrome. His eGFR had dropped considerably compared to the result 2 years earlier (Fig. 5.5).

Because of the apparent suddenness of these complications, a renal biopsy was performed.

It showed typical features of diabetic nephropathy (Figs. 5.6 and 5.7).

The ACE inhibitor ramipril was started, at a modest dose of 5 mg daily. He had not previously taken this class of drug.

Over the following month, the rate of loss of albumin in his urine reduced to levels that could be matched by synthesis in his liver. As a result his serum albumin returned to normal, i.e. he was no longer nephrotic.

The rate of decline in his eGFR slowed dramatically, from 30 ml/min/1.73 m^2/year to 8 ml/min/1.73 m^2/year (Fig 5.8).

He eventually reached end-stage kidney failure and had a combined kidney and pancreas transplant, which transformed his health.

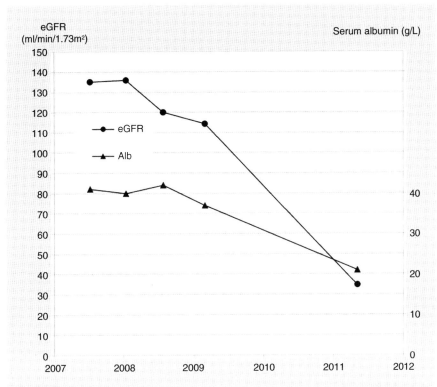

Fig. 5.5 Rapid decline in GFR, 30 ml/min/1.73 m²/year, and drop in serum albumin due to diabetic nephropathy with nephrotic syndrome

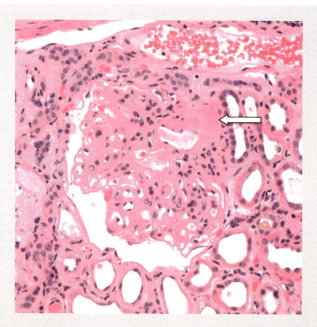

Fig. 5.6 Typical changes of diabetic nephropathy: diffuse glomerulosclerosis and hyalinosis. The walls of the glomerular capillaries are thickened and the mesangium is expanded. There is a nodular deposit of hyaline material at the vascular pole of the glomerulus (*arrow*). Haematoxylin and eosin ×200

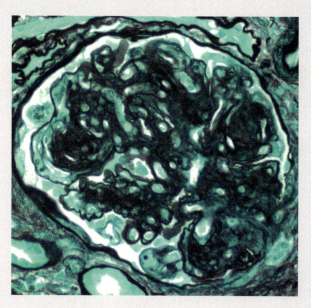

Fig. 5.7 Diffuse glomerular sclerosis of diabetes with Kimmelstiel-Wilson nodules, thickening of the glomerular basement membrane and focal hyalinosis. Silver ×200

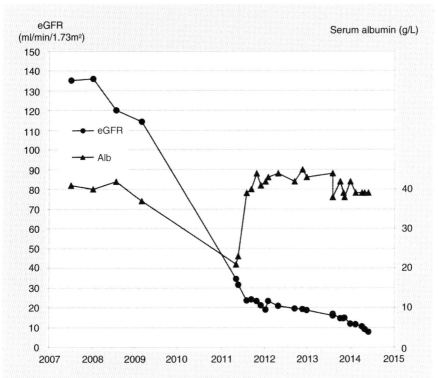

Fig. 5.8 Slowing in the rate of decline in eGFR to 8 ml/min/1.73 m²/year with restoration in serum albumin to normal with ACE inhibitor treatment started in 2011

Atherosclerosis

Patients with cardiovascular disease, such as angina, myocardial infarction or stroke, are likely to have atherosclerosis affecting the renal arterial circulation. There may be a stenosis of one or more renal arteries or diffuse narrowing of the intrarenal arterial tree (see Figs. 5.9 and 5.10).

Renal Artery Stenosis

Renal artery stenosis often causes high blood pressure and reduced kidney function. Less commonly it causes sudden pulmonary oedema despite left ventricular function being well preserved – 'flash' pulmonary oedema.

The degree of loss of kidney function is not proportional to the degree of narrowing of the renal artery. However, as the artery becomes completely occluded, GFR declines (Fig. 5.11).

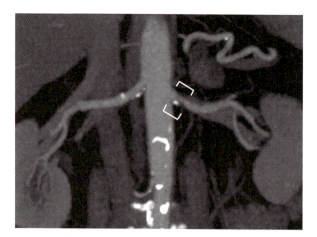

Fig. 5.9 CT angiogram of the abdominal vessels showing a left renal artery stenosis – image taken in the arterial phase. Contrast reveals the blood flowing in the arteries and veins. There are calcified atherosclerotic plaques in the aorta, renal arteries and other vessels. The calcium is in the wall of the arteries which is otherwise not seen and so appears outside the blood in the lumen. There is a narrowing in the lumen near the origin of the left renal artery at the site of a calcified plaque (*brackets*). The left kidney appears smaller than the right

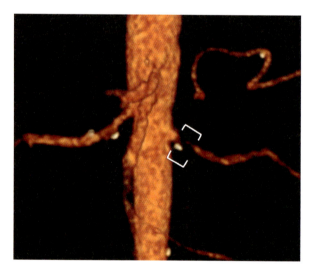

Fig. 5.10 3D reconstruction of the CT scan in Fig 5.9 showing the stenosis more clearly (*brackets*). The column of blood in the left renal artery is narrower than in the right

In the early days of interventional radiology there were some small studies and case series of patients with stenosis of the renal arteries undergoing angioplasty and recovering kidney function (see Fig. 5.12). This led to the hope that angioplasty and stenting of narrowed but not occluded renal arteries would improve blood pressure and halt the decline of kidney function.

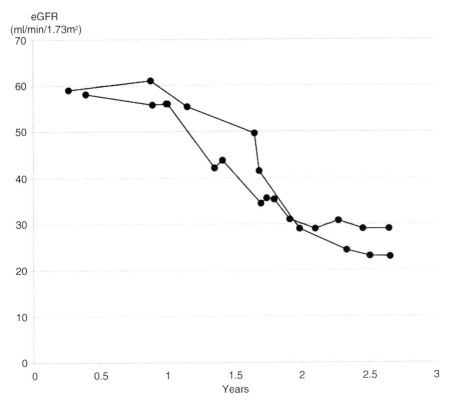

Fig. 5.11 eGFR graphs from two patients with peripheral vascular disease affecting their lower limbs. Their eGFR fell by half over 1 year. In both patients, imaging showed that one kidney had atrophied due to complete occlusion of the renal artery

Unfortunately, a number of clinical trials have since shown that angioplasty and stenting of atherosclerotic renal artery stenosis does not improve kidney function and most patients continue to require antihypertensive drugs [8].

Atherosclerosis of the renal artery is usually associated with more widespread disease of smaller renal arteries and with glomerulosclerosis. Widening of the stenosed renal artery does not improve the more distal disease. It also carries the risk of damaging the arterial wall, causing cholesterol crystal embolisation to the kidney or occluding the artery completely (see Patient 5.3). The procedure is now reserved for patients with flash pulmonary oedema, rapidly worsening kidney function or high blood pressure that cannot be controlled by medication.

The renal arteries can be narrowed by a non-atherosclerotic disease – fibromuscular dysplasia. This is much less common, affects women between 40 and 60 years of age and often involves the carotid arteries [9]. It usually presents with headache and hypertension that cannot be controlled with medication. It rarely causes loss of kidney function. Unlike atherosclerotic disease, it responds well to angioplasty or surgery.

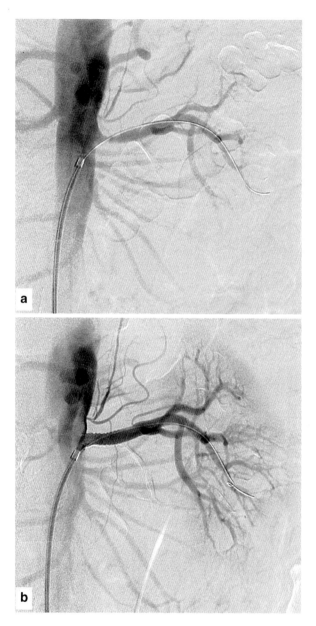

Fig. 5.12 Arteriograms showing a catheter in the left renal artery (**a**). Following balloon angioplasty, a stent has been deployed (**b**). The arterial blood flow to the kidney appears to have improved

Cholesterol Crystal Embolisation (Atheroembolic Disease)

Passing a catheter along an atheromatous artery, such as in a coronary angiogram, carries a risk of destabilising atheromatous plaques. If they lie above the renal arteries, cholesterol crystals are carried downstream to the kidneys where they lodge in the glomeruli. The kidney damage usually progresses over a few weeks or months as cholesterol crystals are repeatedly released into the circulation and a foreign body reaction to the crystals causes further occlusion of the vessel lumen (Fig. 5.13). Less often, massive embolism causes acute kidney injury due to renal infarction (see Fig. 15.4).

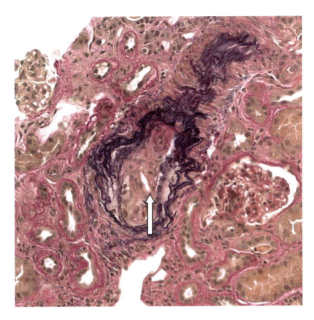

Fig. 5.13 A cholesterol crystal embolism in a small renal artery. The elastic lamina of the artery is stained black. The cholesterol crystal has been dissolved by the processing of the specimen, leaving a cleft (*arrow*). The crystal has stimulated a foreign body reaction with giant cells, occluding the artery. Elastic Van Gieson ×200

Patient 5.3: Cholesterol Crystal Embolisation

Mrs Simpson, aged 86, was admitted as an emergency with chest pain. An ECG showed ST elevation in the inferior leads. Coronary angiography via the right femoral artery showed a stenosis of the left circumflex artery which was stented. Two days later she had another episode of chest pain with ST elevation in leads I, II and V6. Repeat coronary angiography showed a sub-acute stent thrombosis. This was treated with balloon angioplasty and dual anti-platelet therapy using aspirin and ticagrelor. A CT scan showed an atheromatous aorta with a 4.5 cm diameter infrarenal aneurysm.

Over the following 3 months her eGFR declined and the full blood count showed eosinophilia (Fig. 5.14).

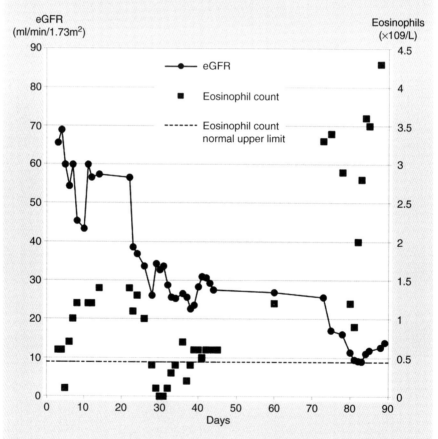

Fig. 5.14 Changes in eGFR and eosinophil count following two coronary angiography procedures

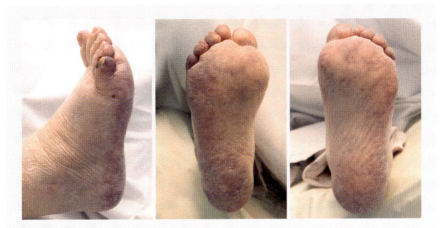

Fig. 5.15 Typical appearances of 'trash feet' due to cholesterol crystal embolisation

Complement C3 was low (0.61, normal range 0.83–1.93); C4 was normal (see Sect. "Complement C3 and C4" in page 202). CRP was modestly elevated (maximum 68 mg/L), in parallel with the eosinophil count. Autoantibodies were not present. Her urine contained no protein, blood, white cells or casts. All these features are consistent with cholesterol crystal embolisation to the kidneys.

She developed a dusky rash over her feet and a painful necrotic little toe (Fig. 5.15). Peripheral pulses were normal. The appearances are characteristic of cholesterol embolisation – so called 'trash feet' with 'blue toe syndrome' and livedo reticularis, a blue network-like discolouration.

The very high eosinophil count and low complement C3 suggested that the kidney disease was linked to an inflammatory response to the crystals.

Chronic Infection and Inflammation

Long-term stimulation of the immune system can lead to a range of glomerular diseases.

Chronic bacterial infections (e.g. tuberculosis, bronchiectasis and osteomyelitis) and inflammatory diseases (e.g. rheumatoid arthritis and Crohn's disease) stimulate the production of acute-phase proteins including serum amyloid A protein. Over years, this protein can accumulate in tissues such as blood vessels, nerves and the kidney to cause AA-amyloidosis. Glomerular involvement manifests as heavy proteinuria or the nephrotic syndrome (see Sect. "Amyloidosis" in page 200).

Chronic viral infections can cause specific glomerular diseases. Chronic hepatitis B infection is associated with membranous nephropathy and mesangiocapillary glomerulonephritis (also called membranoproliferative glomerulonephritis).

Persistence of hepatitis C virus can stimulate B-lymphocytes to produce mixed cryoglobulins that are deposited in capillaries including the glomerulus. This is associated with a vasculitic skin rash and the nephritic syndrome, with fibrinoid necrosis of glomeruli (see Sect. "Complement C3 and C4" in page 202) [10].

HIV-associated nephropathy (HIVAN) can present with nephrotic syndrome or renal failure. Renal biopsy usually shows focal segmental glomerulosclerosis (FSGS) although other histological changes have been reported [11]. The mechanism differs from hepatitis viruses in that the HIV damages the podocytes, causing proteinuria, nephrotic syndrome and glomerulosclerosis, and tubular cells causing renal failure. Before highly active antiretroviral therapy became available, HIVAN progressed rapidly to end-stage kidney disease. This outcome can usually be prevented if proteinuria or reduced eGFR are detected early.

References

1. Raymond NT, Paul O'Hare J, Bellary S, Kumar S, Jones A, Barnett AH, UKADS Study Group. Comparative risk of microalbuminuria and proteinuria in UK residents of south Asian and white European ethnic background with type 2 diabetes: a report from UKADS. Curr Med Res Opin. 2011;27 Suppl 3:47–55. doi:10.1185/03007995.2011.614937. http://informahealth-care.com/doi/abs/10.1185/03007995.2011.614937.
2. Kriz W, Lemley KV. A potential role for mechanical forces in the detachment of podocytes and the progression of CKD. J Am Soc Nephrol. 2015;26:258–69. doi:10.1681/ASN.2014030278. http://jasn.asnjournals.org/content/26/2/258.full.pdf+html.
3. de Boer IH, DCCT/EDIC Research Group. Kidney disease and related findings in the diabetes control and complications trial/epidemiology of diabetes interventions and complications study. Diabetes Care. 2014;37(1):24–30. doi:10.2337/dc13-2113. http://care.diabetesjournals.org/content/37/1/24.full.
4. Coca SG, Ismail-Beigi F, Haq N, Krumholz HM, Parikh CR. Role of intensive glucose control in development of renal end points in type 2 diabetes mellitus: systematic review and meta-analysis intensive glucose control in type 2 diabetes. Arch Intern Med. 2012;172(10):761–9. doi:10.1001/archinternmed.2011.2230. http://archinte.jamanetwork.com/article.aspx?articleid=1170041.
5. Papademetriou V, Lovato L, Doumas M, Nylen E, Mottl A, Cohen RM, Applegate WB, Puntakee Z, Yale JF, Cushman WC, for the ACCORD Study Group. Chronic kidney disease and intensive glycemic control increase cardiovascular risk in patients with type 2 diabetes. Kidney Int. 2015;87:649–59. doi:10.1038/ki.2014.296. http://www.nature.com/ki/journal/v87/n3/full/ki2014296a.html.
6. Gregg EW, Li Y, Wang J, Burrows NR, Ali MK, Rolka D, Williams DE, Geiss L. Changes in diabetes-related complications in the United States, 1990–2010. N Engl J Med. 2014;370:1514–23. doi:10.1056/NEJMoa1310799. http://www.nejm.org/doi/full/10.1056/NEJMx140023.
7. Andrésdóttir G, Jensen ML, Carstensen B, Parving HH, Hovind P, Hansen TW, Rossing P. Improved prognosis of diabetic nephropathy in type 1 diabetes. Kidney Int. 2014;87:417–26. doi: 10.1038/ki.2014.206. http://www.nature.com/ki/journal/v87/n2/abs/ki2014206a.html
8. Jennings CG, Houston JG, Severn A, Bell S, Mackenzie IS, MacDonald TM. Renal artery stenosis—when to screen, what to stent? Curr Atheroc Rep. 2014;16(6):416. doi:10.1007/s11883-014-0416-2. http://link.springer.com/article/10.1007/s11883-014-0416-2/fulltext.html.
9. Escárcega RO, Mathur M, Franco JJ, Alkhouli M, Patel C, Singh K, Bashir R, Patil P. Nonatherosclerotic obstructive vascular diseases of the mesenteric and renal arteries. Clin

Cardiol. 2014;37(11):700–6. doi:10.1002/clc.22305. Epub 2014 Aug 6. http://onlinelibrary.wiley.com/doi/10.1002/clc.22305/pdf.

10. Perico N, Cattaneo D, Bikbov B, Remuzzi G. Hepatitis C Infection and Chronic Renal Diseases. Clin J Am Soc Nephrol. 2009;4(1):207–20. doi:10.2215/CJN.03710708. http://cjasn.asnjournals.org/content/4/1/207.full.

11. Phair J, Palella F. Renal disease in HIV-infected individuals. Curr Opin HIV AIDS. 2011;6(4):285–9. doi:10.1097/COH.0b013e3283476bc3. http://www.ncbi.nlm.nih.gov/pmc/articles/PMC3266688/.

Chapter 6
Are You Pregnant or Planning a Pregnancy?

How Pregnancy Affects the Kidneys and Vice Versa

Abstract In this chapter we explain:

- How to do a risk assessment when planning a pregnancy
- How kidney function changes during pregnancy
- How pregnancy can affect kidney disease
- How kidney disease can affect the outcomes of a pregnancy

Pregnancy in a woman with kidney disease poses risks to both the baby and the mother [1]. These issues can be a significant emotional burden [2].

Risks to the Baby

Overall, the risk of a worse outcome for the baby is more than doubled in women with CKD [3].

Before the pregnancy, drugs that may damage the developing foetus should be reviewed. Drugs commonly used in patients with kidney disease that may be teratogenic include angiotensin-converting enzyme inhibitors, angiotensin II receptor blockers, and immunosuppressive drugs such as mycophenolate. The risk of teratogenicity must be weighed against the risk posed to the mother by stopping the drug [4].

Risks to the Mother

The GFR of normal kidneys increases by 50 % over the first 3 months of a pregnancy (Fig. 6.1). In someone with a well-functioning kidney transplant the GFR will increase by up to this amount, proving that this effect is not mediated by the kidney's nerve supply. If a pregnant woman shows no fall in serum creatinine this is a sign that her nephrons are unable to 'hyperfilter' and she is likely to have underlying chronic kidney disease.

© Springer International Publishing Switzerland 2016
H. Rayner et al., *Understanding Kidney Diseases*,
DOI 10.1007/978-3-319-23458-8_6

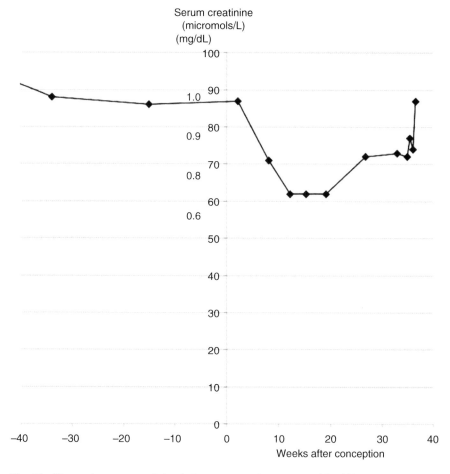

Fig. 6.1 Changes in serum creatinine during pregnancy in a woman with a kidney transplant. The baby was delivered by caesarean section. The last data point is the serum creatinine measured the day after delivery

Hyperfiltration due to pregnancy can damage already diseased glomeruli. The risk increases in proportion to the stage of CKD before pregnancy, whatever the cause of the kidney disease.

If the eGFR is more than 60 ml/min/1.73 m^2 the outlook is good, including with a well functioning transplant. With hypertension or proteinuria there is an increased risk of pre-eclampsia and loss of kidney function. Women with vesico-ureteric reflux have an increased risk of urinary tract infections during pregnancy and may benefit from daily prophylactic antibiotics.

If the eGFR is less than 40 ml/min/1.73 m^2 and there is heavy proteinuria – more than 1 g per day, i.e. protein: creatinine ratio >100 mg/mmol (1000 mg/g) – the rate of decline in GFR is accelerated by pregnancy and the time to end-stage kidney failure shortened [5].

With CKD stages 4 and 5, the likelihood of becoming pregnant is significantly reduced as ovulation is irregular or absent. If conception does occur, the foetus usually does not grow at the normal rate and is either born early or stillborn. Successful pregnancy is a rare but wonderful event in women on dialysis.

Pre-Eclampsia

Pregnancy itself can cause kidney disease, a condition called pre-eclampsia. This presents with hypertension, peripheral oedema and proteinuria, usually in the last 6 weeks of pregnancy. If it presents earlier than 34 weeks the outcomes are worse. The clinical severity of the kidney disease can vary from just hypertension and proteinuria to severe acute kidney injury requiring dialysis due to thrombotic thrombocytopaenic purpura (TTP).

The primary cause of pre-eclampsia is an ischaemic dysfunctional placenta that releases so-called anti-angiogenic factors into the mother's circulation. These factors damage vascular endothelial cells.

The risk of pre-eclampsia is higher in first and twin pregnancies where the level of anti-angiogenic factors is higher, and in women with hypertension, diabetes and obesity where the endothelial cells are more susceptible to these factors. Antiplatelet therapy with low-dose aspirin (75 mg daily) protects the endothelium and reduces the risk of pre-eclampsia by 10 % [6].

In women who have had pre-eclampsia in a previous pregnancy the risk of it recurring is at least 15 %. This increases to over 50 % with increasing severity of the previous episode.

Proteinuria usually clears after the pregnancy. If it is still present after 3 months, another kidney disease may be present. Pre-eclampsia increases the risk of long-term hypertension by up to four times and doubles the risk of ischaemic heart disease, stroke and venous thromboembolism.

Patient 6.1: Assessing the Risk of Pregnancy in a Woman with Chronic Kidney Disease

Christine attended the renal clinic with her new partner at the age of 25. She was under follow up for reflux nephropathy, which she had inherited from her mother. She was desperate to have another baby.

In her first pregnancy 5 years previously she had had pre-eclampsia requiring an emergency caesarian section. During that pregnancy, her GFR had increased only slightly and had dropped during the episode of pre-eclampsia (Fig. 6.2).

Since then it had recovered and the proteinuria had returned to trace on dipstick testing. She was feeling well, not diabetic and had a body mass index of 22 kg/m^2. She was taking the calcium channel blocker amlodipine for high blood pressure that was well controlled.

The following factors that increase the risk of pre-eclampsia were discussed:

- Age older than 40
- First pregnancy
- History of pre-eclampsia
- New paternity
- Interval between pregnancies of less than 2 or more than 10 years
- Multiple pregnancy
- Obesity
- Chronic conditions – high blood pressure, migraine, diabetes, kidney disease, thrombophilia, SLE

Everyone agreed that the risks to her and her baby were acceptable. A urine specimen was sent for culture and she was referred to the renal-antenatal clinic for follow up. She was delighted.

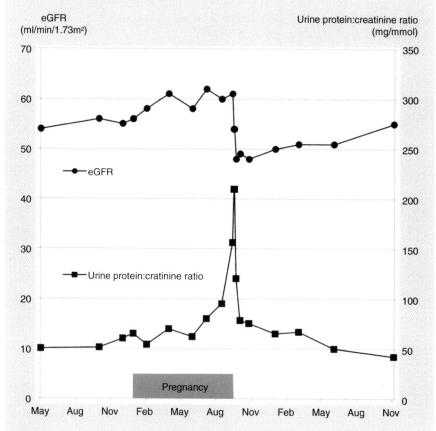

Fig. 6.2 The effect of pregnancy on eGFR and urine protein excretion in a lady with reflux nephropathy. Increasing proteinuria culminated in pre-eclampsia

References

1. Palma-Reis I, Vais A, Nelson-Piercy C, Banerjee A. Renal disease and hypertension in pregnancy. Clin Med. 2013;13:57–62. doi:10.7861/ clinmedicine.13-1-57. http://www.clinmed.rcpjournal.org/content/13/1/57.full.

2. Tong A, Jesudason S, Craig JC, Winkelmayer WC. Perspectives on pregnancy in women with chronic kidney disease: systematic review of qualitative studies. Nephrol Dial Transplant. 2015;30(4):652–61. doi:10.1093/ndt/gfu378. http://ndt.oxfordjournals.org/content/30/4/652.abstract.

3. Nevis IF, Reitsma A, Dominic A, et al. Pregnancy outcomes in women with chronic kidney disease: a systematic review. Clin J Am Soc Nephrol. 2011;6(11):2587–98. doi:10.2215/CJN.10841210. http://www.ncbi.nlm.nih.gov/pmc/articles/PMC3359575.

4. Li DK, Yang C, Andrade S, Tavares V, Ferber JR. Maternal exposure to angiotensin converting enzyme inhibitors in the first trimester and risk of malformations in offspring: a retrospective cohort study. BMJ. 2011;343:d5931. doi:10.1136/bmj.d5931. http://www.bmj.com/content/343/bmj.d5931.

5. Imbasciati E, Gregorini G, Cabiddu G, Gammaro L, Ambroso G, Del Giudice A, Ravani P. Pregnancy in CKD stages 3 to 5: fetal and maternal outcomes. Am J Kidney Dis. 2007;49:753–62. http://www.ajkd.org/article/S0272-6386(07)00692-0/abstract.

6. Askie LM, Duley L, Henderson-Smart DJ, Stewart LA, PARIS Collaborative Group. Antiplatelet agents for prevention of pre-eclampsia: a meta-analysis of individual patient data. Lancet. 2007;369(9575):1791–8. http://www.ncbi.nlm.nih.gov/pubmed/17512048.

Chapter 7
What Is Your Family History?

The Molecular Genetics of Inherited Kidney Diseases

Abstract In this chapter we explain:

- How to draw a family pedigree
- Genetic disorders of the glomerulus and tubules
- Current understanding of cystic kidney diseases
- How vesico-ureteric reflux can be associated with kidney disease

It is well known that some kidney diseases are inherited. It is less well known that someone with a family history of kidney failure has double the normal adult risk of kidney disease *from a different cause*. Their risk of developing chronic kidney disease between 10 and 19 years of age is six times greater [1]. So it is important to ask about any family history of kidney disease and to document the family in a pedigree chart.

Our understanding of the environmental and genetic factors that lead to this increased risk is advancing rapidly. With modern molecular techniques, genetic testing is relatively simple. However, interpretation of the results and the implications they have for someone's physical and psychological health can be more complex.

Knowing that you have inherited a kidney condition may allow you to prepare psychologically and physically for kidney failure. Alternatively it may cause prolonged anxiety about an uncertain prognosis. It may affect your ability to obtain insurance or a mortgage. Informing other family members that they may be at risk and advising whether or not they should be genetically tested is a delicate matter.

If someone has a disease caused by a mutation in a single gene, the predictive value of the mutation, the penetrance, is nearly 100 %. However, the disease may appear at different ages and with different severity. Furthermore, some single-gene diseases vary due to interaction between the abnormal disease gene and a mutation in a modifier gene.

Diseases caused by multiple mutations on different genes are much more common. They have a variable phenotype and are more affected by environmental factors. Genome-wide association studies have identified genes that confer an increased risk for hypertension and diabetic nephropathy, as well as vesico-ureteric reflux, focal

© Springer International Publishing Switzerland 2016
H. Rayner et al., *Understanding Kidney Diseases*,
DOI 10.1007/978-3-319-23458-8_7

segmental glomerulosclerosis (FSGS) and atypical haemolytic uraemic syndrome (aHUS) (see Sect. "Kidney disease linked to causes of anaemia" in page 176) [2].

Genetic abnormalities are like experiments of nature. They have helped us to understand how the kidneys work at a molecular level. We will describe the more common disorders in sequence along the nephron from the glomerulus to the ureter.

The Glomerular Filtration Barrier

Alport Syndrome

Cecil Alport described a syndrome of hereditary nephritis with haematuria and deafness in a British family in 1927 [3]. He thought the nephritis was due to an infection but we now know that it and the deafness are due to a mutation of one of the type IV collagen genes. The abnormal collagen disrupts the structure of membranes in the glomerulus (see Fig. 7.1) and in the organ of Corti in the cochlea.

Alport reported that: "The male members of a family tend to develop nephritis and deafness and do not as a rule survive. The females have deafness and haematuria and live to old age." The type IV alpha 5 collagen gene is located on the X-chromosome, explaining why males are severely affected whereas female heterozygotes are less so.

The presentation of nephritis in males can vary. As Alport reported: "The last couple of cases are interesting evidence of the variations in the course of nephritis. The kidneys of two members of the same family were attacked, apparently by the same organism, at the same time, and under exactly the same conditions. The elder brother contracted acute nephritis, which cleared up completely; the younger developed parenchymatous nephritis, passing into small white kidney, and ending in death."

Alport did not refer to the eye abnormalities that can accompany the syndrome: a misshapen lens (anterior lenticonus) and abnormal colouration of the retina. These rarely lead to loss of vision [4].

A number of conditions have been described within the Alport syndrome family, involving mutations of genes coding for different protein chains that together form type IV collagen. They are mostly X-linked recessive. Some have autosomal recessive inheritance – homozygotes have the syndrome whereas heterozygote carriers are unaffected or have thin glomerular basement membrane nephropathy (see Patient 11.1). A small number show autosomal dominant inheritance, heterozygotes being affected.

Congential Nephrotic Syndrome

Numerous genetic abnormalities, both dominant and recessive, have been described in children with congenital nephrotic syndrome. The age of onset depends upon the gene affected and whether one or both alleles are affected. If the presentation is before 3 months of age, the cause is invariably genetic [5]. The nephrotic syndrome is steroid-resistant and often progresses to renal failure (see Patient 9.1).

The gene mutations lead to abnormal proteins in the basement membrane or the podocytes and have helped to identify the role of these proteins in the glomerular filtration barrier. For example, in the Finnish type of congenital nephrotic syndrome there is an abnormality of nephrin, a transmembrane protein in the slit diaphragm between the podocyte foot processes. Other causes are mutations in the genes coding for laminin and podocin (Fig. 7.2).

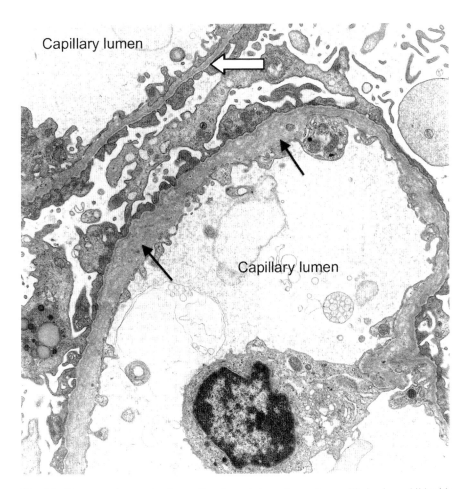

Fig. 7.1 Electron micrograph of a section through two glomerular capillaries in a child with Alport syndrome. The glomerular basement membrane in one capillary is abnormally thin (*white arrow*). The other is abnormally thick and the arrangement of collagen fibres is disorganised (*black arrows*) showing a 'basket-weave' pattern

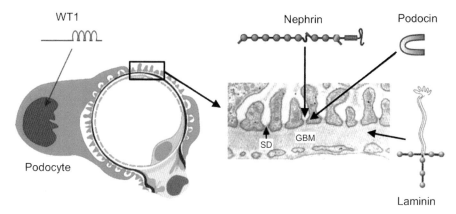

Fig. 7.2 Cross-section of a glomerular capillary (*left*) and electron microscopy image of a normal capillary wall (*right*). WT1 is a transcription factor important for podocyte function. Nephrin is a major component of the slit diaphragm (*SD*) connecting podocyte foot processes. Podocin is an adapter protein located intracellularly in the SD area. Laminin is a major structural protein of the glomerular basement membrane (*GBM*). Genetic mutations in these proteins lead to congenital nephrotic syndrome (From Jalanko [5])

The Tubules

Figure 7.3 summarises the main genetic diseases affecting the nephron.

The Proximal Tubule

The majority of the reabsorption and secretion of solutes occurs in the proximal tubule [7]. The surface area of the tubule is maximised by the brush border micro-villi on the epithelial cell surface. The main features of the genetic disorders that disrupt solute transport are polyuria and the loss of electrolytes, sugar or amino acids into the urine. Table 7.1 describes some of the more common disorders.

The Loop of Henle

The loop of Henle is the part of the nephron which enables urine to be concentrated and water conserved [8]. In the thick ascending limb, sodium, potassium and chloride ions are reabsorbed by transporter proteins but water cannot follow [9]. Ions are trapped within the interstitium of the medulla, creating a concentration gradient. The hyperosmolar environment in the deep medulla draws water out of the collecting duct.

Mutations of the genes that code for transporter proteins lead to a condition called Bartter syndrome. The effects are similar to the action of loop diuretics such

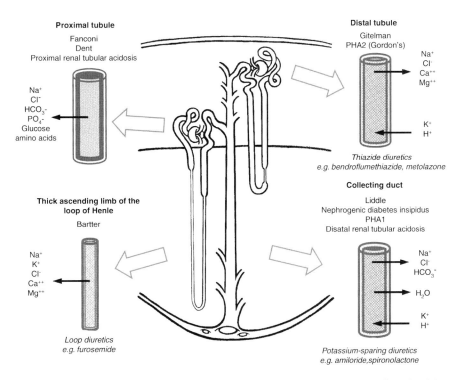

Fig. 7.3 Genetic diseases of the nephron, the normal transport functions that are affected and the sites of action of the main classes of diuretics [6]

as furosemide, which blocks the transport of sodium, potassium and chloride into the cells of the thick ascending limb.

Abnormally large amounts of sodium ions flow from the loop of Henle into the distal tubule where they are reabsorbed in exchange for potassium and hydrogen ions. Hence the patient, usually a child, has polyuria, hypovolaemia, hypokalaemia, hypochloraemia and metabolic alkalosis.

Because calcium and magnesium normally are reabsorbed with sodium and chloride in the thick ascending limb, there is also hypercalciuria and hypomagnesaemia.

There are five types of Bartter syndrome with varying renal and extrarenal manifestations [10].

The Distal Tubule

The main function of the distal convoluted tubule is the reabsorption of sodium and chloride, as well as some calcium and magnesium [11]. The sodium/chloride transporter is blocked by thiazide diuretics such as bendroflumethiazide. An autosomal

Table 7.1 Genetic disorders of the proximal tubule, their mode of inheritance and clinical consequences

Solute	Gene symbol	Gene product(s)	Inheritance	Disorder	Consequence
Glucose	SLC5A1 SLC5A2	Na/Glu cotransporter SGLT1 SGLT2	AR	Renal glycosuria	Positive urine dipstick test for glucose
Amino acids e.g. cystine	CSNU1 SLC7A9	amino acid transporter	AR	Cystinuria	Cysteine stones
Bicarbonate	CA2 SLCA4A	Carbonic anhydrase NaHCO$_3$ cotransporter	AR	Proximal (type 2)	Metabolic acidosis
Multiple solutes	CLCN5	Cl− channel	XR	Dent type 1 disease: Fanconi syndrome (uricosuria, glycosuria, phosphaturia, aminoaciduria, low molecular weight proteinuria) and proximal renal tubular acidosis	Nephrocalcinosis, stones, osteomalacia, rickets
Phosphate	PHEX SLC34A3	Endopeptidase which regulates FGF23 NaP-cotransporter	XD AR	Hypophosphataemic rickets	Phosphaturia, vitamin D resistant rickets

AR autosomal recessive, *AD* autosomal dominant, *XR* X-linked recessive, *XD* X-linked dominant

recessive mutation that leads to loss of its function causes similar effects, a condition called Gitelman syndrome [10]. Compared to Bartter syndrome, the salt loss and volume contraction is less severe. The condition usually presents in older children and adults when hypokalaemia and metabolic alkalosis are detected incidentally on a U&E result. In contrast to Bartter syndrome and in line with the effect of thiazides, calcium excretion is reduced.

The opposite of Gitelman syndrome is Gordon's syndrome (pseudohypoaldosteronism type 2, PHA2), an autosomal dominant condition in which the sodium/chloride transporter is overactivated. Excessive sodium reabsorption results in high blood pressure. Reduced potassium and hydrogen ion excretion leads to hyperkalaemia and metabolic acidosis. Thiazide diuretics effectively counteract the abnormalities in Gordon's syndrome.

The Collecting Duct

The collecting duct has two cell types:

- principal cells which reabsorb salt and water, secrete potassium, and control the concentration of the urine [12]
- intercalated cells which regulate acid–base balance by secreting hydrogen ions and adjusting bicarbonate [13]

The principal cells contain membrane channels that selectively allow sodium and water to enter the cell and potassium to leave. Sodium is then pumped out through the basal membrane by the Na/K ATPase. An autosomal dominant mutation prevents the epithelial sodium channel being removed from the cell membrane leading to increased absorption of sodium and excretion of potassium and H+. This results in high blood pressure, hypokalaemia and metabolic alkalosis – Liddle syndrome – which is counteracted by amiloride, a potassium-sparing diuretic.

The sodium and potassium channels and the Na/K ATPase in the basal membrane are regulated by aldosterone. Its overall effect is to increase sodium reabsorption and potassium excretion. Mutations of the gene coding for the sodium channel make it unable to respond to aldosterone – pseudohypoaldosteronism type 1 (PHA1). This results in the opposite of Liddle syndrome – salt wasting, hyperkalaemia and acidosis, like Addison's disease.

The water channel (aquaporin 2) is controlled by the antidiuretic hormone, vasopressin, acting on its receptor. Mutations in the genes that code for the vasopressin receptor or for the water channel lead to hereditary nephrogenic diabetes insipidus. Because the ability to concentrate the urine is lost, the patients have polyuria and nocturia. Urine osmolality is low and plasma osmolality inappropriately raised. This stimulates thirst, leading to polydipsia and preventing severe hypernatraemia.

The intercalated cells break down carbonic acid to H^+ and bicarbonate via a reaction catalyzed by carbonic anhydrase. The H^+ ions are actively pumped into the urine by an H^+ ATPase. The bicarbonate ions are carried to the blood by a Cl^-/

HCO_3^- anion exchanger. Genetic mutations causing loss of function of either of these mechanisms leads to distal (type 1 RTA). The H^+ ATPase is also present in the inner ear, hence autosomal recessive mutations cause distal RTA with congenital sensorineural deafness.

The inappropriately alkaline urine in distal RTA leads to the precipitation of calcium in the urine as stones or within the kidney tissue as nephrocalcinosis. In adults, this syndrome is more commonly an acquired defect associated with autoimmune diseases.

Uromodulin

Formerly known as Tamm-Horsfall protein, uromodulin is the most abundant protein in normal urine. Its function is not well understood [14]. It is secreted by the thick ascending limb of the loop of Henle and the distal tubule, where it modulates the sodium and potassium channels. It may also protect against urinary tract infections, ischaemia and stone formation.

Mutations in the uromodulin (UMOD) gene lead to Uromodulin Kidney Disease, an autosomal-dominant condition only fully characterised in the last decade. Genome-wide association studies have also identified the UMOD gene as a risk factor for CKD and hypertension.

Mutations in the UMOD gene alter the structure of uromodulin, preventing its release from the kidney cells and allowing leakage back into the interstitial space around the tubules. In this location uromodulin has an inflammatory effect, leading to interstitial nephritis and fibrosis. End-stage kidney failure is reached between 30 and 60 years of age (Patient 7.1).

Affected kidneys are also unable to excrete uric acid normally. This leads to hyperuricaemia and the early onset of gout.

Patient 7.1: Uromodulin Kidney Disease

Nick had a kidney transplant 15 years ago. At that time the cause of his kidney failure was unclear. He had severe hypertension throughout his 20's and had not been at all keen on having a kidney biopsy. His late mother had gout from the age of 16 followed by severe hypertension, renal failure and a transplant. A renal biopsy had shown normal glomeruli, hypertensive changes in the vessels and some atrophy of the collecting tubules.

Nick's sister also had severe hypertension and renal failure and had sadly died from complications after a kidney transplant. Neither Nick nor his sister had gout.

On this occasion, Nick attended clinic with his son, aged 19, who was having occasional attacks of gout. His blood pressure was 159/107 mmHg and his eGFR was 53 ml/min/1.73 m^2. His urine contained no blood or protein. His serum urate was 769 micromol/L (normal range 200–430).

The association of teenage gout, hypertension and progressive CKD pointed to uromodulin kidney disease. The family had samples taken for genetic testing, which confirmed that Nick and his son and daughter had all inherited a mutation of the uromodulin gene.

Nick's family pedigree chart is shown in Fig. 7.4.

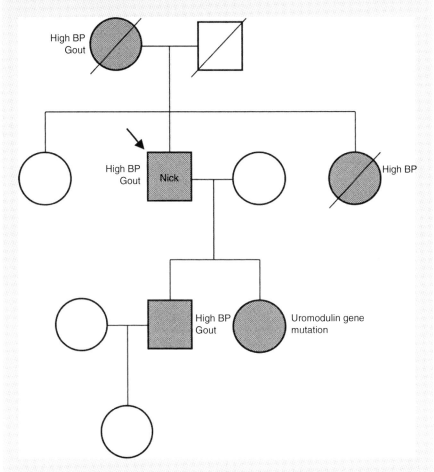

Fig. 7.4 Nick's uromodulin kidney disease family pedigree, consistent with autosomal dominant inheritance

Cystic Kidney Diseases

Cysts feature in a range of genetic disorders and can develop from all segments of the nephron. They vary in size from small, e.g. medullary sponge kidney (a condition recently recognised as inherited) [15, 16] to large, e.g. autosomal dominant polycystic kidney disease.

The cysts develop from the proliferation of tubular cells forming a bulge in the normal tubule. The bulge breaks off from the lumen to form a cyst surrounded by fibrous tissue. Instead of absorbing solutes, the cells lining the cyst secrete fluid into the lumen making it enlarge.

Over the age of 50 years, it is very common for normal kidneys to form a few simple cysts. At least one cyst is present in more than 20 % of people aged over 70 years. [17]. They can reach a large size but are rarely of any clinical significance (see Sect. "Appearances in kidney disease" in page 215).

There is evidence that abnormal function of the primary cilia in tubular cells underlies all the genetic cystic conditions, so they have been called the ciliopathies [18]. Each cell in the body has one primary cilium, equivalent to the flagellum on motile single cell organisms [19]. As fluid flows along the tubule the cilia are moved and the epithelial cell senses the direction and rate of flow. They may also sense the chemical composition of the tubular fluid.

Movement of the cilia triggers the release of chemical messengers which control the transport functions of tubular epithelial cells. Malfunction of the cilia stops the epithelial cells detecting flow and removes the control of normal cell division, allowing them to proliferate and dilate the tubule. The membrane transport processes are disrupted and the cells secrete fluid into the lumen to enlarge the cyst (Fig. 7.5).

The three commonest inherited cystic kidney diseases are nephronophthisis, autosomal recessive (ARPKD) and autosomal dominant polycystic kidney disease (ADPKD). Nephronophthisis is the commonest genetic cause of kidney failure in childhood. The kidneys are normal sized or small and cysts form near the border of the cortex and medulla. It is caused by mutations in a range of recessive genes and can be associated with extra-renal abnormalities, such as in Bardet-Biedl syndrome [20].

ARPKD is due to mutations in a large gene that codes for the protein fibrocystin/polyductin. This protein is located on the primary cilium of the tubular epithelial cell and plays a critical role in controlling the division of cells into two rather than into multiple daughter cells [21]. Despite having the same mutation, the clinical presentation may vary – cysts forming in utero or in the neonatal period. The protein is also found in the cilia of bile duct cholangiocytes and some older children present with symptoms caused by liver disease.

ADPKD is due to a mutation in one of the genes PKD1 or PKD2; 85 % of patients have the PKD1 mutation. The genes code for polycystin, a protein that controls the function of cilia. It is thought that in early life the normal PKD allele of the heterozygote controls cell division. In adulthood, the normal allele may undergo a somatic mutation – a 'second hit' – and a clone of cells divides to form a cyst (see Fig. 7.5). Alternatively, the production of polycystin by some cells may fall below the threshold level required to control cilia, allowing unregulated cell proliferation.

Criteria have been agreed to help distinguish incidental simple cysts found on ultrasound from the early stages of ADPKD (Fig. 7.6) [23]. Cysts can also develop in the liver, pancreas and spleen (Fig. 7.7). Weakness of the arterial walls of intracranial arteries can lead to berry aneurysms and sub-arachnoid haemorrhage. Weakness of the heart valve apparatus can cause mitral valve prolapse.

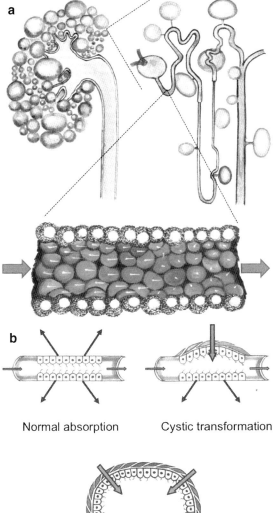

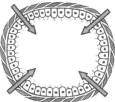

Fig. 7.5 How cysts are thought to form from tubules in genetic polycystic kidney disease. (**a**) Three levels of magnification: the whole kidney; a single nephron; a cutaway view of a tubule as seen under scanning electron microscopy. The cells on the left of the tubule have normal cilia that are aligned with the flow of tubular fluid. On the *right* the cilia are abnormal and do not correctly sense the flow of fluid. (**b**) The normal tubule reabsorbs fluid and electrolytes. The abnormal cells change from an absorptive to a secretory phenotype and proliferate to form a bulge in the tubule, which separates off as a cyst. The remaining nephron ceases to function. Secretion enlarges the cyst and fibroblasts proliferate around it [22]

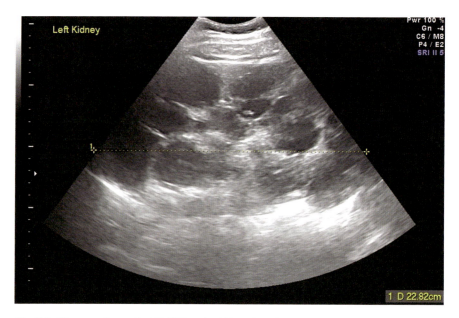

Fig. 7.6 Ultrasound scan in ADPKD – the kidney is enlarged and contains multiple simple cysts

The progression of kidney failure in ADPKD is related to the growth of cysts. When the cyst breaks off, the remaining nephron ceases to function. As the cysts enlarge, surrounding nephrons are compressed and obstructed. Interventions such as blood pressure control have a less beneficial effect on the decline in kidney function than in glomerular diseases where there is proteinuria. However, hypertension often develops early in the disease and warrants treatment for its cardiovascular benefits.

A patient's prognosis can be estimated from the size of the kidneys. If they are longer than 16.5 cm on an ultrasound scan the patient is more likely to develop stage 3 CKD [24]. Treatments that may slow the growth rate have been tried, with interesting results reported using the vasporesssin antagonist tolvaptan in adults and the HMG-CoA reductase inhibitor pravastatin in childhood [25].

Kidney Tumours

A number of autosomal dominant mutations lead to the formation of benign and malignant kidney tumours. Familial papillary cell carcinomas result from a mutation causing overactivity of the MET proto-oncogene. The kidney tumours may be one part of a characteristic syndrome of abnormalities caused by mutations of tumour suppressor genes; for example tuberous sclerosis [26], von-Hippel-Lindau disease [27] and Wilms-tumor-aniridia syndrome [28].

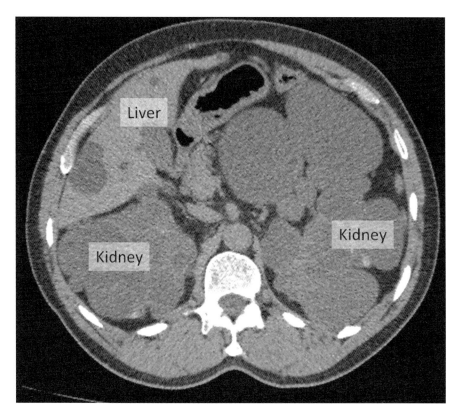

Fig. 7.7 CT scan with intravenous contrast from the same patient as in Fig. 7.6. The kidneys are grossly enlarged by multiple cysts, which are also present in the liver

The Lower Urinary Tract

The junction between the ureter and bladder normally acts as a valve, preventing the flow of urine back up the ureter during micturition when the pressure within the bladder increases. If this valve is incompetent, vesico-ureteric reflux (VUR) occurs [29].

The embryological development of the junction between the ureter and bladder is a complex process involving chemical signaling to control the differentiation and organization of cells. This process may be affected by genetic abnormalities and by mechanical forces acting on the developing structures.

When VUR is familial, inheritance is usually autosomal dominant, although recessive and X-linked inheritances have been reported. The wide range in the severity of the damage, from asymptomatic to end-stage kidney disease, suggests that a variety of underlying abnormalities can lead to VUR.

VUR can be an isolated finding or associated with abnormalities such as posterior urethral valves or ureterocele. VUR can also be part of a multiorgan malformation syndrome – congenital abnormalities of the kidney and ureteric tract (CAKUT) [30]. For example, the urogenital sinus may persist in females so that the urethra and vagina do not have separate openings. The vagina or uterus becomes distended and compresses the urethra, increasing pressure in the bladder and causing VUR. Ureteric obstruction in the developing embryo in utero causes hydronephrosis and dysplasia of the kidneys with a reduced number of functioning nephrons at birth. As much of the kidney parenchymal damage occurs in utero, end-stage kidney disease is not easily prevented (see Patient 7.2).

VUR can reduce in severity or resolve completely during childhood [31]. Surgery to reduce the ureteric reflux is no more effective than prophylactic antibiotics in reducing the risk of kidney scarring [32]. A recent randomised trial showed that prophylactic antibiotic treatment also does not prevent scarring but does halve the rate of urine infection [33].

Patient 7.2: Complex Vesico-Ureteric Reflux (VUR)
Aisha was the first of twin girls born by emergency caesarean section at 28 weeks gestation because her mother had pre-eclampsia. An antenatal ultra-sound scan had shown bilateral renal pelvic dilatation. A scan soon after birth was normal because urine volume is low in the first few days.

Aisha was treated with prophylactic trimethoprim. Despite this, during the first 3 months she had septicaemia from an *Enterococcus faecalis* urine infection. Later, a suprapubic urine specimen cultured a pure growth of *Escherichia coli*. She responded well to antibiotics.

Her serum creatinine was 144 micromol/L (1.63 mg/dL) compared to the normal range for her age of 18–51 micromol/L. A DMSA isotope scan (see Sect. " Isotope renography" in page 223) was performed at 3 months of age to measure the relative function of her two kidneys. It showed 75 % of total function in the right kidney, 25 % in the left (Fig. 7.8).

A micturating cystogram was performed at 5 months of age to image the anatomy of her ureters and bladder. It showed severe bilateral vesico-ureteric reflux (Fig. 7.9).

A MAG 3 renogram was performed to track the flow of urine down the urinary tract (see Sect. "Isotope renography" in page 223). It showed very poor ureteric drainage from both kidneys (Fig. 7.10).

An ultrasound scan showed both kidneys to be echogenic (see Sect. "Ultrasound" in page 215). There was bilateral hydronephrosis and hydro-ureter with a very dilated right lower ureter (Fig. 7.11). The bladder was tra-beculated, indicating muscle hypertrophy due to bladder outlet obstruction.

Cystoscopy revealed a urogenital sinus and bilateral paraureteric diverticu-lae caused by the pressure from bladder outlet obstruction. To relieve the obstruction, the bladder was opened to the anterior abdominal wall – a vesi-costomy. At age 8 the vesicostomy was closed, the bladder enlarged using redundant ureteric tissue and a Mitrofanoff fistula fashioned using her appen-dix to allow the bladder to be catheterized directly (Fig. 7.12).

Aisha's blood pressure was raised from the age of 4 years. Despite treatment with the ACE inhibitor enalapril, her GFR progressively declined due to hyper-filtration of the remaining nephrons. She received a kidney transplant at age 11.

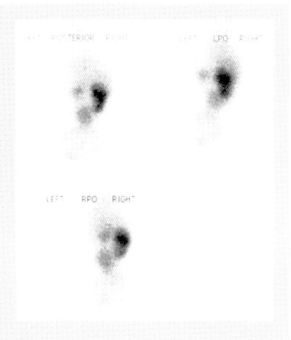

Fig. 7.8 DMSA scan from three viewing angles – posterior, left posterior-oblique (*LPO*) and right posterior-oblique (*RPO*). The right kidney has taken up much more isotope than the left

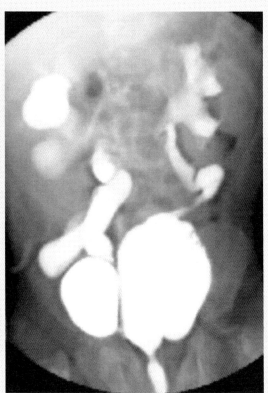

Fig. 7.9 Micturating cystogram showing severe bilateral vesico-ureteric reflux

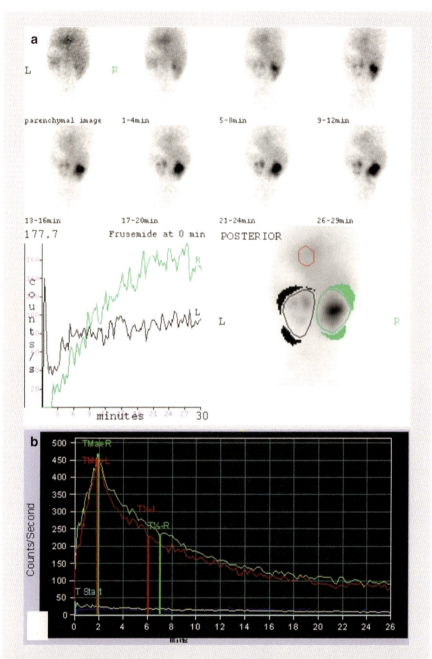

Fig. 7.10 (**a**) MAG3 renogram from Aisha. There is delayed uptake of isotope by the kidneys, measured as counts/s of radioactivity. The right kidney trace peaks at 27 min (normal <6 min). The left kidney reaches a lower level than the right due to its relatively worse function. There is no decline from either kidney within 30 min indicating obstruction to urinary flow (normal T½ < 15 min). (**b**) A normal renogram for comparison showing symmetrical uptake and excretion of the isotope; TMax = 2 min, T½ *left* = 6 min, T½ *right* = 7 min

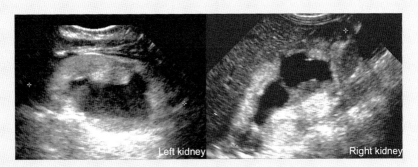

Fig. 7.11 Ultrasound scan of the kidneys showing echogenic kidneys with bilateral hydro-nephrosis and hydroureter

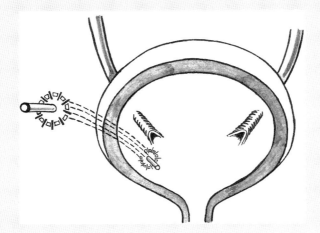

Fig. 7.12 Diagramatic representation of a Mitrofanoff fistula with a catheter in place

References

1. Akrawi DS, Li X, Sundquist J, Sundquist K, Zöller B. Familial risks of kidney failure in Sweden: a nationwide family study. PLoS One. 2014;9(11):e113353. doi:10.1371/journal.pone.0113353. eCollection 2014. http://www.ncbi.nlm.nih.gov/pmc/articles/PMC4244139/.
2. Hildebrandt F. Genetic kidney diseases. Lancet. 2010;375(9722):1287–95. doi:10.1016/S0140-6736(10)60236-X. http://www.ncbi.nlm.nih.gov/pmc/articles/PMC2898711/.
3. Alport AC. Hereditary familial congenital haemorrhagic nephritis. BMJ. 1927;1(3454):504–6. doi:10.1136/bmj.1.3454.504. http://www.ncbi.nlm.nih.gov/pmc/articles/PMC2454341/.
4. Savige J, Sheth S, Leys A, Nicholson A, Mack HG, Colville D. Ocular features in Alport syndrome: pathogenesis and clinical significance. Clin J Am Soc Nephrol. 2015;10(4):703–9. doi:10.2215/CJN.10581014. http://cjasn.asnjournals.org/content/early/2015/01/30/CJN.10581014.abstract.
5. Jalanko H. Congenital nephrotic syndrome. Pediatr Nephrol. 2009;24(11):2121–8. doi:10.1007/s00467-007-0633-9. http://www.ncbi.nlm.nih.gov/pmc/articles/PMC2753773.
6. Walsh SB, Unwin RJ. Renal tubular disorders. Clin Med. 2012;12:476–9. doi:10.7861/clinmedicine.12-5-476. http://www.clinmed.rcpjournal.org/content/12/5/476.full.

7. Curthoys NP, Moe OW. Proximal tubule function and response to acidosis. Clin J Am Soc Nephrol. 2014;9(9):1627–38. doi:10.2215/CJN.10391012. http://cjasn.asnjournals.org/content/9/9/1627.full.

8. Dantzler WH, Layton AT, Layton HE, Pannabecker TL. Urine-concentrating mechanism in the inner medulla: function of the thin limbs of the loops of henle. Clin J Am Soc Nephrol. 2014;9(10):1781–9. doi:10.2215/CJN.08750812. http://cjasn.asnjournals.org/content/9/10/1781.full.

9. Mount DB. Thick ascending limb of the loop of henle. Clin J Am Soc Nephrol. 2014;9(11):1974–86. doi:10.2215/CJN.04480413. http://cjasn.asnjournals.org/content/9/11/1974.full.

10. Fremont OT, Chan JC. Understanding Bartter syndrome and Gitelman syndrome. World J Pediatr. 2012;8(1):25–30. doi:10.1007/s12519-012-0333-9. Epub 2012 Jan 27. http://link.springer.com/article/10.1007%2Fs12519-012-0333-9.

11. Subramanya AR, Ellison DH. Distal convoluted tubule. Clin J Am Soc Nephrol. 2014;9(12):2147–63. doi:10.2215/CJN.05920613. http://cjasn.asnjournals.org/content/9/12/2147.full.

12. Pearce D, Soundararajan R, Trimpert C, Kashlan OB, Deen PMT, Kohan DE. Collecting duct principal cell transport processes and their regulation. Clin J Am Soc Nephrol. 2015;10(1):135–46. doi:10.2215/CJN.05760513. http://cjasn.asnjournals.org/content/early/2014/05/28/CJN.05760513.full.

13. Roy A, Al-bataineh MM, Pastor-Soler NM. Collecting duct intercalated cell function and regulation. Clin J Am Soc Nephrol. 2015;10(2):305–24. doi:10.2215/CJN.08880914. http://cjasn.asnjournals.org/content/early/2015/01/27/CJN.08880914.full?sid=796c6bff-f0fc-48ed-9a74-2b31e165e316.

14. Rampoldi L, Scolari F, Amoroso A, Ghiggeri G, Devuyst O. The rediscovery of uromodulin (Tamm-Horsfall protein): from tubulointerstitial nephropathy to chronic kidney disease. Kidney Int. 2011;80(4):338–47. doi:10.1038/ki.2011.134. Epub 2011 Jun 8.]. http://www.ncbi.nlm.nih.gov/pubmed/21654721.

15. Goldfarb DS. Evidence for inheritance of medullary sponge kidney. Kidney Int. 2013;83:193–6. doi:10.1038/ki.2012.417. http://www.nature.com/ki/journal/v83/n2/full/ki2012417a.html.

16. Fabris A, Lupo A, Ferraro PM, Anglani F, Pei Y, Danza FM, Gambaro G. Familial clustering of medullary sponge kidney is autosomal dominant with reduced penetrance and variable expressivity. Kidney Int. 2013;83:272–7. doi:10.1038/ki.2012.378. http://www.nature.com/ki/journal/v83/n2/full/ki2012378a.html.

17. Ravine D, Gibson RN, Donlan J, Sheffield LJ. An ultrasound renal cyst prevalence survey: specificity data for inherited renal cystic diseases. Am J Kidney Dis. 1993;22(6):803–7. http://www.ncbi.nlm.nih.gov/pubmed/8250026.

18. Davenport JR, Yoder BK. An incredible decade for the primary cilium: a look at a once-forgotten organelle. Am J Physiol Renal Physiol. 2005;289(6):F1159–69. doi:10.1152/ajprenal.00118.2005. http://ajprenal.physiology.org/content/289/6/F1159.

19. Pluznick JL, Caplan MJ. Chemical and physical sensors in the regulation of renal function. Clin J Am Soc Nephrol. 2015;10(9):1626–3. doi:10.2215/CJN.00730114. http://cjasn.asnjournals.org/content/early/2014/10/02/CJN.00730114.full.

20. Zaghloul NA, Katsanis N. Mechanistic insights into Bardet-Biedl syndrome, a model ciliopathy. J Clin Invest. 2009;119(3):428–37. doi:10.1172/JCI37041. http://www.jci.org/articles/view/37041.

21. Zhang J, Wu M, Wang S, Shah JV, Wilson PD, Zhou J. Polycystic kidney disease protein fibrocystin localizes to the mitotic spindle and regulates spindle bipolarity. Hum Mol Genet. 2010;19(17):3306–19. doi:10.1093/hmg/ddq233. first published online June 16, 2010; http://hmg.oxfordjournals.org/content/19/17/3306.full.

22. Avner ED, McDonough AA, Sweeney WE. Transport, cilia, and PKD: must we in (cyst) on interrelationships? Am J Physiol Cell Physiol. 2012;302(10):C1434–5. doi:10.1152/ajpcell.00070.2012. http://www.ncbi.nlm.nih.gov/pmc/articles/PMC3362002/.

23. Pei Y, Obaji J, Dupuis A, Paterson AD, Magistroni R, Dicks E, Ravine D. Unified criteria for ultrasonographic diagnosis of ADPKD. J Am Soc Nephrol: JASN. 2009;20(1):205–12. doi:10.1681/ASN.2008050507. http://www.ncbi.nlm.nih.gov/pmc/articles/PMC2615723.

24. Bhutani H, Smith V, Rahbari-Oskoui F, Mittal A, Grantham JJ, Torres VE, Mrug M, Bae KT, Wu Z, Ge Y, Landslittel D, Gibbs P, O'Neill WC, Chapman AB. A comparison of ultrasound and magnetic resonance imaging shows that kidney length predicts chronic kidney disease in autosomal dominant polycystic kidney disease. Kidney Int. 2015;88(1):146–51. doi:10.1038/ki.2015.71. Epub 2015 Apr. http://www.nature.com/ki/journal/v88/n1/full/ki201571a.html.

25. Ong ACM, Devuyst O, Knebelmann B, Walz G. Autosomal dominant polycystic kidney disease: the changing face of clinical management. Lancet. 2015;385(1993):2002. http://www.thelancet.com/journals/lancet/article/PIIS0140-6736(15)60907-2/abstract.

26. The Tuberous Sclerosis Association http://www.tuberous-sclerosis.org.

27. Von Hippel-Lindau disease http://www.patient.co.uk/doctor/von-hippel-lindau-disease.

28. International WAGR Syndrome Association http://www.wagr.org.

29. Williams G, Fletcher JT, Alexander SI, Craig JC. Vesicoureteral reflux. J Am Soc Nephrol. 2008;19:847–62. doi:10.1681/ASN.2007020245. published ahead of print March 5, 2008. http://jasn.asnjournals.org/content/19/5/847.abstract.

30. Song R, Yosypiv IV. Genetics of congenital anomalies of the kidney and urinary tract. Pediatr Nephrol. 2011;26(3):353–64. doi:10.1007/s00467-010-1629-4. Epub 2010 Aug 27. http://link.springer.com/article/10.1007%2Fs00467-010-1629-4.

31. Edwards D, Normand ICS, Prescod N, Smellie JM. Disappearance of vesicoureteric reflux during long-term prophylaxis of urinary tract infection in children. Br Med J. 1977;2:285–8. http://www.bmj.com/content/2/6082/285.

32. Birmingham Reflux Study Group. Prospective trial of operative versus non-operative treatment of severe vesicoureteric reflux in children: five years' observation. Br Med J (Clin Res Ed). 1987;295:237–41. http://www.bmj.com/content/295/6592/237.

33. The RIVUR Trial Investigators. Antimicrobial prophylaxis for children with vesicoureteral reflux. N Engl J Med. 2014;370:2367–76. http://www.nejm.org/doi/full/10.1056/NEJMoa1401811#t=articleTop.

Chapter 8
What Have You Been Taking?

Nephrotoxicity from Medications and Other Chemicals

Abstract In this chapter we explain:

- How ACE inhibitors and angiotensin receptor blockers work
- How drugs can be nephrotoxic through
  - Vasoconstriction
  - Tubulotoxicity
  - Interstitial inflammation
- MINT cocktails
- The interaction between metformin and kidney function
- Kidney damage due to heroin, cocaine, mushrooms and chemicals

A detailed drug history is a crucial part of the assessment of any patient, especially when kidney disease is suspected. The history must cover the nature of any drugs taken – prescribed or otherwise. The use of alternative remedies derived from plants and animals is increasing worldwide and many are associated with acute kidney injury [1].

Details of each drug, when it was started and stopped, and the doses prescribed and taken should be compared to changes in the patient's kidney function.

Some commonly used drugs can affect kidney function and/or structure, in other words can be nephrotoxic. There are three main mechanisms of injury: ischaemia, tubular toxicity and interstitial inflammation. Injury to the glomerulus is less common [2, 3].

Vasoactive Drugs

For glomerular filtration to occur, blood needs to flow into the glomeruli at an adequate rate and under sufficient pressure to force filtration through the glomerular filtration barrier (see Sect. "Turning blood into urine" in page 1). Vasoactive drugs can affect glomerular filtration by varying vascular resistance and the dynamics of glomerular blood flow.

© Springer International Publishing Switzerland 2016
H. Rayner et al., *Understanding Kidney Diseases*,
DOI 10.1007/978-3-319-23458-8_8

ACE Inhibitors and Angiotensin Receptor Blockers

Angiotensin-II (A-II) constricts the efferent arterioles, increasing the glomerular filtration pressure by restricting the flow of blood out of the glomeruli. The effect of A-II is inhibited by Angiotensin Converting Enzyme (ACE) inhibitors, which block the synthesis of A-II, and Angiotensin Receptor Blockers (ARBs), which inhibit the action of A-II on its receptor (Fig. 8.1). Both classes of drug allow the efferent

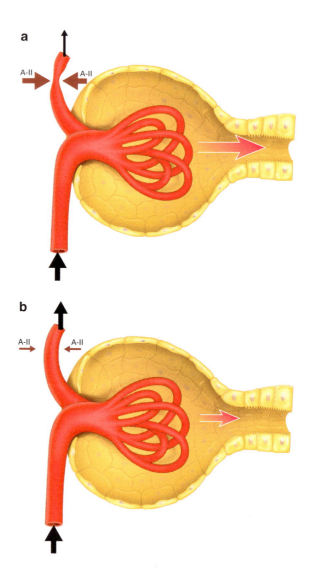

Fig. 8.1 (a) The effect of angiotensin II on glomerular filtration. AII causes vasoconstriction of the efferent arteriole and increases glomerular filtration pressure and rate. (b) Inhibition of AII leads to dilatation of the efferent arteriole, releasing the intra-glomerular pressure and reducing glomerular filtration rate

arterioles to dilate and so lower the glomerular filtration pressure. The drop in GFR is usually small and the reduction in intraglomerular pressure can be beneficial by reducing hydrostatic damage and glomerulosclerosis.

If the pressure in the afferent arteriole is low, glomerular filtration is dependent upon vasoconstriction of the efferent arteriole to maintain intraglomerular pressure. This is the case in someone with poor left ventricular function and low systolic blood pressure or with atherosclerosis of the renal arteries causing a drop in pressure upstream of the glomeruli.

If such a person is given an ACEI or an ARB, there is a risk that the drop in intraglomerular pressure will be clinically significant (Patient 8.1). There is a typical pattern of changes in the laboratory results that helps to identify this effect:

- ↓ eGFR – low glomerular filtration pressure
- ↑ potassium – reduced AII stimulation of aldosterone production, leading to reduced potassium excretion
- ↑ urea-to-creatinine ratio – slow flow of filtrate along the nephron allowing diffusion of urea back into the blood (see Sect. "Serum urea and creatinine – different measures of kidney function" in page 26).

Patient 8.1: Recurrent ACE Inhibitor Nephrotoxicity
Mrs. Blake, aged 72 years, had high blood pressure, proteinuria and diabetes. She was started on the ACE inhibitor lisinopril and her blood pressure became well controlled. Over the following year her eGFR steadily declined and the serum urea and potassium levels rose, suggesting that the ACE inhibitor was the cause (Fig. 8.2). The lisinopril was stopped and her eGFR returned to its previous level. The high blood pressure was controlled with a calcium channel blocker.

Four years later, a doctor unfamiliar with her history reviewed Mrs Blake in the diabetes clinic. This doctor was concerned about the heavy proteinuria and so started ramipril.

Changes in eGFR, urea and potassium repeated the pattern of 4 years previously, this time to more extreme values as her underlying kidney function had worsened (Fig. 8.2).

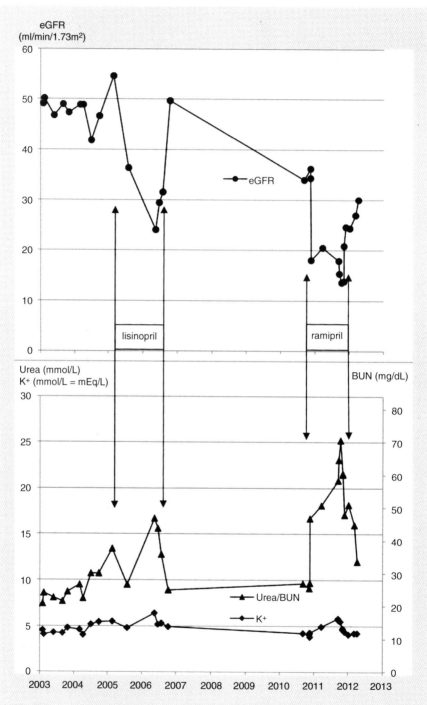

Fig. 8.2 Changes in eGFR, serum urea and serum potassium during repeated periods of ACE inhibitor treatment

Non-steroidal Anti-inflammatory Drugs

Blood flow through kidney arterioles is maintained by vasodilator prostaglandins. Non-steroidal anti-inflammatory drugs (NSAIDs) inhibit cyclo-oxygenase enzymes and reduce the production of prostaglandins. Removing the vasodilator effect of prostaglandins leads to vasoconstriction and a drop in renal blood flow and GFR.

Overdosage of NSAIDs can cause acute kidney injury (Patient 8.2). Normal doses given repeatedly over a prolonged period can lead to permanent damage from ischaemia.

Patient 8.2: NSAID Overdose

John, an 18-year-old musician who suffered from depression, was admitted having taken an overdose of 300 mg seroxat, 700 mg diclofenac and 3.5 g naproxen. His U&E's were normal: creatinine = 103 micromols/L (1.2 mg/dL), eGFR = 87. After a psychiatric assessment, he went home.

Over the next 2 days he became unwell with vomiting and pain in the loins and so returned to hospital. His eGFR had dropped to 50 and continued to decline over the following 3 days (Fig. 8.3). In retrospect, the initial creatinine result had indicated acute kidney injury as 2 years previously it had been 77 micromols/L (0.9 mg/dL). The peak serum creatinine was 287 micromols/L (3.2 mg/dL) making this episode AKI stage 3 (see Table 3.2).

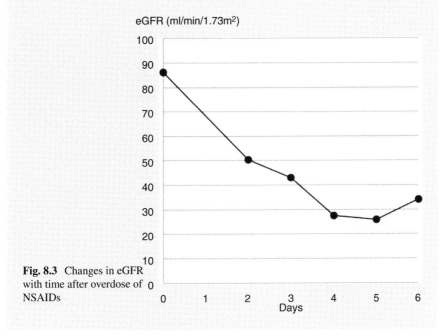

Fig. 8.3 Changes in eGFR with time after overdose of NSAIDs

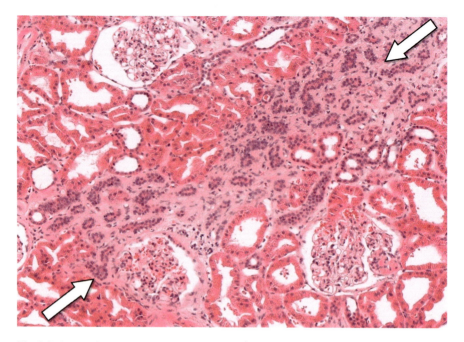

Fig. 8.4 A transplant kidney biopsy showing a band of fibrosis through the interstitium caused by long-term ciclosporin therapy (*arrows*). The glomeruli are normal. Haematoxylin and eosin ×200

Calcineurin Inhibitors – Two Sides of a Coin

Calcineurin inhibitors such ciclosporin and tacrolimus preserve the function of kidney transplants by preventing rejection. Ironically, one of their main side effects is to reduce GFR by vasoconstriction of kidney arterioles. With chronic use, this leads to ischaemic damage and fibrosis, arranged in stripes along the radial distribution of the intrarenal arterioles (Fig. 8.4).

Mixing Vasoactive Drugs to Make MINT Cocktails

The commonest situation causing acute kidney injury is where a number of drugs that alone would not significantly reduce GFR are used together. This has been termed a Multifactorial Iatrogenic NephroToxicity or MINT cocktail .[1]

---

[1] Dr. Es Will, Consultant Nephrologist, St James' University Hospital, Leeds, personal communication 1992.

In patients with diabetes, long-standing hypertension, vascular disease or advanced age, kidney blood supply may be chronically compromised. Combining an ACE inhibitor, which reduces intraglomerular pressure, and a diuretic, which drops plasma volume and thereby renal blood flow, can lead to a marked drop in

Patient 8.3: A MINT Cocktail

Mrs. Kent was admitted as an emergency on 31st October having had a painful swollen right knee for 3 weeks. She had had no fever but her CRP (C-reactive protein) was very high, 237 mg/L, suggesting a septic arthritis. Her urine contained + protein on dipstick testing. Her serum creatinine was 57 micromols/L (0.6 mg/dL).

The large effusion in her knee was aspirated. The fluid was turbid with pus cells but no crystals or organisms. On the afternoon of 1st November she was taken to theatre for an arthroscopy and washout.

Her blood pressure on admission was 126/74 mmHg with a pulse rate of 109 beats per minute but this fell to an average of 100/65 for 12 h prior to the operation. Her blood pressure averaged 80/50 under the 30 min anaesthetic and 100/60 for 12 h following the operation before returning to normal.

Her usual medications were continued including losartan 50 mg once daily for hypertension, and pregabalin 150 mg twice daily and naproxen 500 mg twice daily for pain. She was started on intravenous benzyl penicillin and flucloxacillin.

Here is her medication chart (Fig. 8.5).

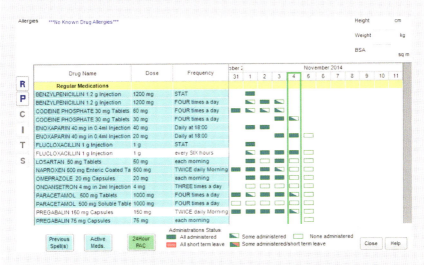

Fig. 8.5 Medication chart for Mrs. Kent documenting the drugs administered following her admission to hospital

The next day she felt better and began physiotherapy. Routine blood tests taken the morning after the operation were reviewed later that day and showed acute kidney injury, serum creatinine = 271 micromols/L (3.1 mg/dL). The next day this had risen to a peak of 459 micromols/L (5.2 mg/dL), AKI stage 3 (see Table 3.2).

Despite a normal blood pressure of 135/78, Mrs Kent felt dizzy and had visual hallucinations in her peripheral vision. This was attributed to the accumulation of pregabalin and codeine, which are normally excreted by the kidneys.

The following medications were stopped: losartan, naproxen, codeine, pregabalin and omeprazole. Intravenous fluids were given, urine volume increased and Mrs Kent went on to make a good recovery. By the time of discharge from hospital, serum creatinine was 108 micromols/L (1.2 mg/dL), eGFR = 48 ml/min/1.73 m², a 50 % drop in GFR compared to before the illness.

GFR (see Patient 8.1). Patients with normal kidneys can suffer acute kidney injury if a sufficient number of nephrotoxic factors are combined (see Patient 8.3).

The insult that leads to acute kidney injury is sometimes predictable, such as a surgical operation. This provides an opportunity for interventions that can protect the kidneys from acute tubular cell damage. One of these is ischaemic preconditioning in which the inherent protective reaction of cells to an insult is used to prepare the kidneys for the subsequent insult of surgery. Ischaemic preconditioning involves inflating a blood pressure cuff on the upper arm to above arterial pressure for 3 min three times, while the patient is under the anesthetic prior to surgery. In patients at high risk of AKI having cardiac surgery, this simple manoeuver reduces the risk of AKI and the need for dialysis after the operation [4]. The effect may be mediated by molecules that temporarily arrest the tubular epithelial cells in the G1 phase of the cell cycle. This protects them from the damaging effects on cell turnover of the second insult.

Tubulotoxic Drugs

Lithium

Lithium carbonate is a highly effective mood-stabilising drug used in the treatment of bipolar disorder. It can restore mental health without the sedative effects of other psychotropic drugs. Unfortunately, in a minority of patients chronic use leads to progressive tubulotoxicity and loss of kidney function, despite careful monitoring of serum drug levels. End stage kidney failure is reached after an average of 20 years' treatment [5].

Lithium is reabsorbed by cells in the collecting duct via the sodium channel. Once inside the cell it can inhibit the effect of vasopressin on the water channel, causing diabetes insipidus. This effect can be reduced by amiloride, which blocks the entry of lithium into the cell via the sodium channel. Lithium also has effects on the parathyroid glands, causing hyperparathyroidism and hypercalcaemia.

When progressive kidney damage due to lithium is detected, the patient is posed a difficult dilemma. Should they stop taking it to avoid further kidney damage, take alternative medications with unpleasant side effects and risk a relapse into mania or depression? Or should they continue the lithium, enjoy continuing stable mental health and risk further damage? Resolving these issues requires close collaboration between the nephrologist, the psychiatrist, the primary care team and the patient.

The decision needs to be made before kidney damage becomes too advanced (see Patient 8.4). The risk that kidney function will continue to decline despite stopping

Patient 8.4: Lithium Nephrotoxicity

Mrs. Ballard had suffered multiple episodes of mania and depression since the age of 25. She started lithium in 1989. It was stopped in 1991 but she relapsed into mania so it was restarted. Her mood then stabilized and she felt well. Serum lithium levels were consistently within the therapeutic range.

By 2008 it was clear her kidney function was declining (Fig. 8.6). Despite the risk of another relapse in her bipolar disorder, she decided to stop lithium and use other antipsychotic and mood stabilizing drugs. The rate of decline in eGFR slowed significantly.

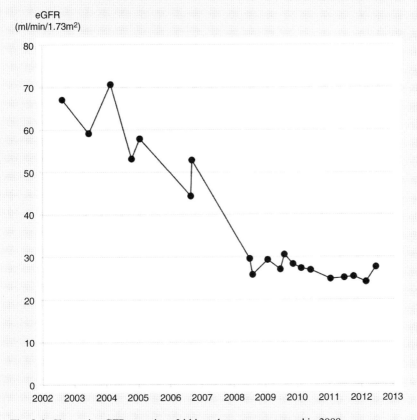

Fig. 8.6 Change in eGFR over time. Lithium therapy was stopped in 2008

lithium increases when eGFR falls below 45 ml/min/1.73 m^2. Stopping lithium at an advanced stage of CKD risks precipitating mental illness at the same time as the patient has the stress of preparing for dialysis or transplantation.

Aminoglycoside Antibiotics – Gentamicin

The antibiotic gentamicin is tubulotoxic as well as ototoxic [6]. Sodium and water reabsorption are affected, especially in the proximal part of the nephron that is exposed to the drug. Urine volume is usually normal or increased and increased amounts of tubular enzymes, aminoacids, glucose, calcium and magnesium are excreted.

Glomerular filtration is reduced by:

- Increased tubulo-glomerular feedback – reduced absorption in the proximal tubule allows more filtrate to reach the distal tubule and the macula densa. This stimulates the release of vasoconstrictors which reduce glomerular filtration and protect against excessive salt and water loss
- Reduction in renal blood flow due to arteriolar vasoconstriction
- Contraction of, and damage to, mesangial cells in the glomeruli
- Obstruction of nephrons with debris from damaged cells, especially in the proximal tubule

The risk of nephrotoxicity increases with the cumulative dose of gentamicin. However, even one dose can have an impact when it is part of a MINT cocktail. Some evidence for this comes from tracking the rate of AKI after orthopaedic surgery in Scottish hospitals. After a change in antibiotic policy from cefuroxime to a combination of flucloxacillin and a single-dose of gentamicin (4 mg/kg) there was a doubling in the rate of AKI [7].

Interstitial Nephritis

Many drugs have the rare side effect of interstitial nephritis – an infiltration of acute inflammatory cells between the nephrons. Examples include antibiotics derived from penicillin and proton pump inhibitors such as omeprazole (Fig. 8.7).

Metformin – Villain or Victim?

The diabetes drug metformin is sometimes mistakenly blamed as being nephrotoxic. This is because it is stopped in patients with reduced GFR and this act is interpreted as meaning that the GFR was being damaged by the drug.

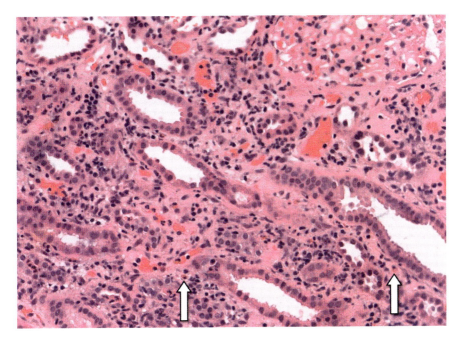

Fig. 8.7 Section of a kidney biopsy from a patient who had been taking omeprazole, showing typical appearances of interstitial nephritis. There is an infiltration of inflammatory cells between the tubules, mainly lymphocytes with some eosinophils *(arrows)*. The glomerulus *(top right)* is normal. Haematoxylin and eosin ×200

In fact metformin is a victim of kidney failure. One of its actions is to increase lactic acid production from pyruvate by reducing pyruvate dehydrogenase activity in the liver. In advanced kidney failure metformin accumulates, leading to potentially fatal lactic acidosis.

Metformin has been used for decades and caution about lactic acidosis is deeply rooted in medical teaching. However, a recent metanalysis of over 200 studies involving 100,000 people suggests that the risk may have been exaggerated [8]. The main factor leading to lactic acidosis in patients taking metformin may be the underlying condition rather than the drug and there may be no increased risk in continuing it, so long as it is stopped when a patient becomes acutely unwell [9].

Kidney Diseases Due to Toxins

Cocaine and Heroin

Use of cocaine and heroin has been associated with the nephrotic syndrome, acute glomerulonephritis, amyloidosis, interstitial nephritis, and rhabdomyolysis (see Patient 11.1: Rhabdomyolysis, myoglobinuria and acute kidney injury) [10]. The kidney damage may be mediated by chronic viral infections such as Hepatitis B, C and HIV and the existence of a specific 'heroin nephropathy' is now questioned. Cocaine is a potent vascoconstrictor and so leads to reduced renal blood flow and GFR. It accelerates atherosclerosis and platelet aggregation and can lead to malignant hypertension.

Mushroom Poisoning

Mushroom poisoning has caused outbreaks of renal failure throughout history and has been blamed for the death of many notable people. Mushrooms of the *Cortinarius* species (the Deadly Webcap) can be confused with edible Chanterelle mushrooms. They cause severe acute kidney injury and permanent renal failure. The toxic effect is due to orellanine, which causes tubular necrosis and interstitial nephritis. Clinical symptoms occur from 3 days to 3 weeks after ingestion. Identifying the spores and detecting the orellanine toxin in leftover mushrooms confirms the diagnosis. Orellanine is detectable by thin-layer chromatography technique in biopsy tissue for up to 6 months. There is no effective antidote [11].

Chemical Poisoning

The following are some of the more common chemicals known to be nephrotoxic:

- Heavy metals – cadmium, lead, mercury
- Melamine – added to baby milk formula
- Ethylene glycol antifreeze
- Glyphosate weed killer

As one of roles of the kidneys is the excretion of toxins, they are especially vulnerable to damage from these chemicals [12].

References

1. Jha V, Rathi M. Natural medicines causing acute kidney injury. Semin Nephrol. 2008;28(4): 416–28. doi:10.1016/j.semnephrol.2008.04.010. http://www.seminarsinnephrology.org/article/S0270-9295(08)00088-0/abstract.
2. Markowitz GS, Bomback AS, Perazella MA. Drug-induced glomerular disease: direct cellular injury. Clin J Am Soc Nephrol. 2015;10(7):1291–9. doi:10.2215/CJN.00860115. http://cjasn.asnjournals.org/content/early/2015/04/10/CJN.00860115.abstract.
3. Hogan JJ, Markowitz GS, Radhakrishnan J. Drug-induced glomerular disease: immune-mediated injury. Clin J Am Soc Nephrol. 2015;10(7):1300–10. doi:10.2215/CJN.01910215. http://cjasn.asnjournals.org/content/early/2015/06/18/CJN.01910215.abstract.

4. Zarbock A, Schmidt C, Van Aken H, Wempe C, Martens S, Zahn, Wolf B, Goebel U, Schwer CI, Rosenberger P, Haeberle H, Görlich D, Kellum JA, Meersch M, for the RenalRIPC Investigators. Effect of remote ischemic preconditioning on kidney injury among high-risk patients undergoing cardiac surgery: a randomized clinical trial. JAMA. 2015. doi:10.1001/jama.2015.4189. http://jama.jamanetwork.com/article.aspx?articleid=2299339

5. Presne C, Fakhouri F, Noël L-H, Stengel B, Even C, Kreis H, Mignon F, Grünfeld J-P. Lithium-induced nephropathy: rate of progression and prognostic factors. Kidney Int. 2003;64:585–92. doi:10.1046/j.1523-1755.2003.00096.x. http://www.nature.com/ki/journal/v64/n2/full/4493918a.html.

6. Lopez-Novoa JM, Quiros Y, Vicente L, Morales AI, Lopez-Hernandez FJ. New insights into the mechanism of aminoglycoside nephrotoxicity: an integrative point of view. Kidney Int. 2011;79:33–45. doi:10.1038/ki.2010.337. http://www.nature.com/ki/journal/v79/n1/full/ki2010337a.html.

7. Bell S, Davey P, Nathwani D, Marwick C, Vadiveloo T, Sneddon J, Patton A, Bennie M, Fleming S, Donnan PT. Risk of AKI with Gentamicin as surgical prophylaxis. J Am Soc Nephrol. 2015;25(11):2625–32. doi:10.1681/ASN.2014010035. http://www.ncbi.nlm.nih.gov/pmc/articles/PMC4214537/.

8. Salpeter SR, Greyber E, Pasternak GA, Salpeter EE. Risk of fatal and nonfatal lactic acidosis with metformin use in type 2 diabetes mellitus. Cochrane Database Syst Rev. 2006;(1):CD002967. http://onlinelibrary.wiley.com/doi/10.1002/14651858.CD002967.pub4/full

9. Metformin associated lactic acidosis. BMJ. 2009; 339. doi: http://dx.doi.org/10.1136/bmj.b3660. (Published 16 Sept 2009). http://www.bmj.com/content/339/bmj.b3660

10. Jaffe JA, Kimmel PL. Chronic nephropathies of cocaine and heroin abuse: a critical review. Clin J Am Soc Nephrol. 2006;1(4):655–67. doi:10.2215/CJN.00300106. http://cjasn.asnjournals.org/content/1/4/655.full.

11. Frank H, Zilker T, Kirchmair M, Eyer F, Haberl B, Tuerkoglu-Raach G, Wessely M, Gröne HJ, Heemann U. Acute renal failure by ingestion of Cortinarius species confounded with psychoactive mushrooms: a case series and literature survey. Clin Nephrol. 2009;71(5):557–62. http://www.dustri.com/nc/journals-in-english/mag/clinical-nephrology/vol/volume-71/issue/may-15.html.

12. Perazella MA. Renal vulnerability to drug toxicity. Clin J Am Soc Nephrol. 2009;4(7):1275–83. doi:10.2215/CJN.02050309. http://cjasn.asnjournals.org/content/4/7/1275.full.

Chapter 9
Height and Weight

The Effects of Kidney Disease on Body Size and Composition

Abstract In this chapter we explain:

- How kidney disease affects children's growth and development
- The role of obesity in kidney disease

Growing Up with Kidney Disease

Chronic kidney disease has a major impact on children's development and quality of life, particularly through its effects on growth. The lower a child's kidney function, the slower will be their rate of growth. As a result, about a third of children with CKD fall below the third percentile for their age and gender. When kidney function is reduced in infancy the effect is even greater.

There is normally rapid growth in head circumference and brain volume during the first year of life. Poor growth is associated with intellectual impairment and learning difficulties. In older children, reduced growth and delayed puberty are associated with worse physical function and increased mortality. Short stature may lead to low self-esteem and emotional difficulties as children grow up to be adults.

An essential part of the care of any child, especially one with kidney disease, is the charting of height, weight and, for infants, head circumference (Patient 9.1).

Patient 9.1: Congenital Nephrotic Syndrome

Rayaan was born to consanguineous parents at term. An ultrasound scan at 20 weeks gestation had shown increased echogenicity of the kidneys. A repeat scan after birth confirmed them to be slightly large and echogenic. Kidney function was normal but serum albumin was low, 17 g/L. A urine dipstick test showed heavy proteinuria confirming congenital nephrotic syndrome (see Sect. "Congential nephrotic syndrome in page 84).

Over the next few days he became progressively more oedematous. He was given the ACE inhibitor captopril and NSAID indomethacin to reduce renal blood flow and urinary protein loss, and was supplemented with daily intravenous infusions of 20 % albumin.

Despite nasogastric feeding, his weight gain over the next three months was very slow and his head circumference barely increased (Fig. 9.1).

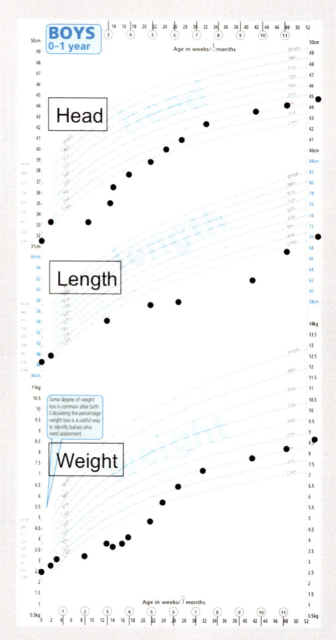

Fig. 9.1 Chart from a boy with congenital nephrotic syndrome showing delayed growth in head circumference, body length and body weight

To further reduce urinary protein loss, one of his kidneys was removed surgically.

Over the next four months his head circumference and then body weight increased rapidly. By 12 months of age, his weight and head circumference were between the 9th and 25th centile and his length was on the 0.4th centile.

Growth failure in kidney disease is mainly due to a functional deficiency of Insulin-like Growth Factor 1 (IGF-1) [1]. Although the serum level of growth hormone is disproportionally high, its stimulatory effect on IGF-1 production by the liver is reduced. Bioactive IGF-1 is reduced and inhibitory IGF binding proteins are increased. The severity of these abnormalities is proportional to the reduction in GFR. Treatment with pharmacological doses of recombinant growth hormone can overcome some of the functional deficiency of IGF-1 (Patient 9.2).

Patient 9.2: Growth Retardation Due to Chronic Kidney Disease
Peter was born with dysplastic kidneys and reduced GFR. Despite nutritional supplements, calcium and vitamin D, his height remained below the 0.4th centile. Recombinant growth hormone injections were started and over the following three years his height velocity increased so that his height crossed the 0.4th centile (Fig. 9.2).

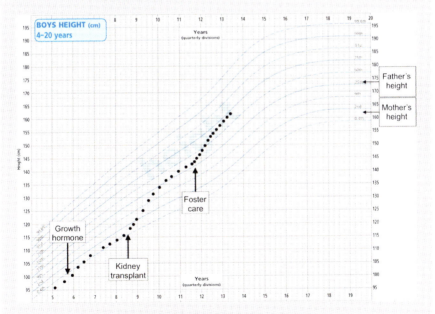

Fig. 9.2 Growth chart from a boy with chronic kidney disease showing the effects of growth hormone, kidney transplantation and improved social circumstances

His renal function continued to decline and at 8.5 years of age he received a live-related kidney transplant. Over the next 18 months his height velocity accelerated so that he crossed the 25th centile for height, consistent with the height of his father.

Sadly, his family life became very difficult and at age 11.5 years he was taken into foster care. He was much happier in this environment; his height velocity increased and he entered puberty just below the 75th centile for height.

As well as these hormonal abnormalities, growth can be affected by poor nutrition, metabolic acidosis, fluid and electrolyte abnormalities, renal bone disease and steroid therapy (Patient 9.3). Disadvantaged social circumstances may compound the medical problems. The most effective treatment is the restoration of normal kidney function with a successful transplant.

Patient 9.3: Growth Retardation and Obesity Due to Steroids
Aneesh attended the paediatric clinic for supervision of his asthma treatment. His height and weight were charted to monitor the effect of inhaled steroids on his growth. Until the age of seven both were increasing along the 50th centile (Fig. 9.3).

He then developed nephrotic syndrome, which is associated with atopy and asthma [2]. Glucocorticoid treatment led to remission of the proteinuria but stimulated his appetite. His weight accelerated and crossed the 75th centile.

During the following two years his nephrotic syndrome relapsed three times, requiring high doses of prednisolone on each occasion. His weight progressively increased, crossing the 91st centile, but his height velocity slowed to below the 50th centile.

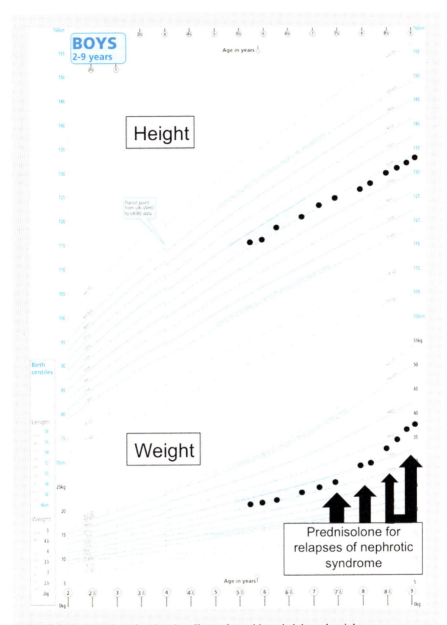

Fig. 9.3 Growth chart showing the effects of steroids on height and weight

Chronic kidney disease leads to a delay in puberty, on average by 2.5 years. When puberty does begin, the pubertal growth spurt may be shortened and less rapid. Bone maturation occurs at the end of puberty. If this is before growth has been completed the child will remain below the predicted height (Patient 9.4).

Patient 9.4: Growth and Puberty
Dominic's kidney disease was not apparent until the age of 15 when he presented acutely unwell with severely impaired kidney function and small shrunken kidneys. He was extremely short for his age and had delayed puberty, his radiological bone age being 4 years less than his chronological age (Fig. 9.4).

He was given recombinant growth hormone with some response in his height. Six months later he received a kidney transplant donated by his mother. Minimal doses of corticosteroid were used to allow maximum growth.

Because his bones were immature he was able to grow at a very rapid rate. By the time he completed his pubertal growth spurt he had reached a height between that of his parents.

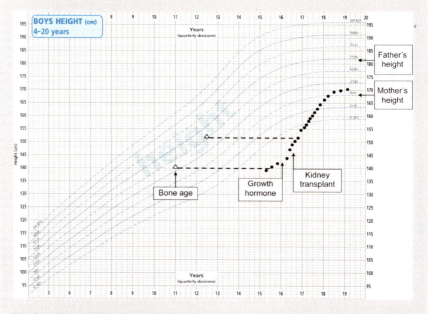

Fig. 9.4 Growth chart showing a delayed pubertal growth spurt in a boy with chronic kidney disease treated with growth hormone and a kidney transplant

Some children with CKD may appear younger than their age because of their reduced growth and delayed puberty. In their teenage years others may treat them as children rather than young adults, delaying their emotional development.

Transitional Care

There comes a time when medical care needs to be transferred from the paediatric team to an adult kidney service. This can be a stressful experience for the young adult and his parents, especially if the support network built up over many years is lost. The break in continuity combined with the challenges of adolescence can precipitate a deterioration in health, for example an increased risk of kidney transplant rejection.

The age when the transfer should occur is best determined by the emotional maturity of the child and the readiness of the family. Ideally, the transition is made through a joint clinic provided by both paediatric and adult teams in an environment designed around the needs of teenagers [3].

Obesity and Risk

As an adult, being overweight or obese indirectly increases the risk of kidney disease through high blood pressure, diabetes and cancer. Obesity is also associated with proteinuria due to focal segmental glomerulosclerosis [4]. In people with diabetes, long-term weight loss achieved through reduced food intake and increased exercise reduces the risk of a decline in eGFR and an increase in albuminuria [5].

In patients on dialysis the usual association of obesity with mortality is not found; instead, increasing body mass index (BMI) is associated with progressively lower mortality. The greater nutritional reserve of overweight dialysis patients may protect them during episodes of acute illness [6].

Obesity is associated with an increased risk of complications after transplant surgery, creating a theoretical dilemma for overweight dialysis patients on the transplant waiting list. Losing weight may improve the outcomes for the transplant but worsen them while they remain on dialysis. Many transplant centres apply a maximum acceptable BMI for inclusion on the waiting list to minimise the risk associated with the transplant procedure and maximise the survival chances of the graft.

References

1. Tönshoff B, Kiepe D, Ciarmatori S. Growth hormone/insulin-like growth factor system in children with chronic renal failure. Pediatr Nephrol. 2005;20(3):279. http://link.springer.com/article/10.1007%2Fs00467-005-1821-0.
2. Abdel-Hafez M, Shimada M, Lee PY, Johnson RJ, Garin EH. Idiopathic nephrotic Syndrome and atopy: is there a common link? Am J Kidney Dis. 2009;54(5):945–53. doi:10.1053/j.ajkd.2009.03.019. http://www.ncbi.nlm.nih.gov/pmc/articles/PMC2895907.
3. Watson AR, Warady BA. Transition from pediatric to adult-centered care. Dial Transplant. 2011;40(4):156–8. http://onlinelibrary.wiley.com/enhanced/doi/10.1002/dat.20557/.
4. Mallamaci F, Tripepi G. Obesity and CKD progression: hard facts on fat CKD patients. Nephrol Dial Transplant. 2013;28 Suppl 4:iv105–8. doi:10.1093/ndt/gft391. http://ndt.oxfordjournals.org/content/28/suppl_4/iv105.full.pdf.

5. The Look AHEAD Research Group. Effect of a long-term behavioural weight loss intervention on nephropathy in overweight or obese adults with type 2 diabetes: a secondary analysis of the Look AHEAD randomised clinical trial. Lancet Diab Endocrinol. 2014;2(10):801–9.
6. Pifer TB, Mccullough KP, Port FK, Goodkin DA, Maroni BJ, Held PJ, Young EW. Mortality risk in hemodialysis patients and changes in nutritional indicators: DOPPS. Kidney Int. 2002;62:2238–45. doi:10.1046/j.1523-1755.2002.00658.x. http://www.nature.com/ki/journal/v62/n6/full/4493347a.html.

Chapter 10
Blood Pressure

A Common Theme in Kidney Disease

Abstract In this chapter we explain:

- The benefits of patients managing their own blood pressure
- Diurnal rhythm in blood pressure
- The importance of night-time blood pressure
- The role of blood pressure in progressive kidney disease

Blood pressure is a simple and informative physiological measurement. Inexpensive and accurate automated arm cuff meters are available in chemist shops. Wrist meters are not recommended; they can give inaccurate readings.

Blood pressure measured in the surgery or clinic may be affected by the 'white coat' effect. This can increase the systolic blood pressure by 30 mmHg or more, even in patients who are not overtly anxious. The size of the effect increases with the underlying blood pressure, making clinic readings of limited value for monitoring blood pressure control. Home blood pressure readings are much more useful.

Patients should be instructed in how to adjust their blood pressure treatment in response to their home readings. In a randomised trial comparing self-monitoring and self-titration of antihypertensive medication versus usual primary care, systolic blood pressure was on average 9 mmHg lower in the self-managing group after 12 months, without any increase in side effects. This big difference would probably lead to a significant improvement in longer-term outcomes [1].

There is often a difference in blood pressure between the two arms [2]. This is more common in people with hypertension, diabetes and chronic kidney disease and is associated with an increased risk of cardiovascular and all-cause mortality. It is recommended to use the higher reading to guide treatment decisions.

Patients with a difference in blood pressure between the two arms of more than 35 mmHg may have an atherosclerotic stenosis of one subclavian artery. Smaller inequalities are more likely to be due to differences in the stiffness of the arteries in the arm than to localised stenotic lesions.

© Springer International Publishing Switzerland 2016
H. Rayner et al., *Understanding Kidney Diseases*,
DOI 10.1007/978-3-319-23458-8_10

Diurnal Variation in Blood Pressure

Blood pressure normally follows a pattern across the 24 h cycle – the diurnal rhythm. It dips before sleep then rises before wakening (Fig. 10.1).

In people with chronic kidney disease, this nocturnal dipping pattern is often lost; a non-dipping pattern being increasingly common as GFR decreases (Fig. 10.2).

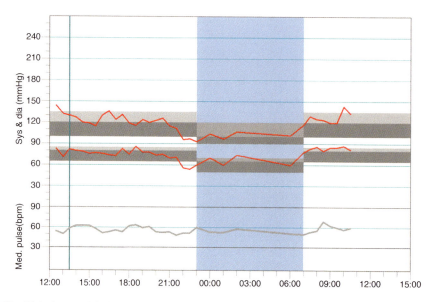

Fig. 10.1   A normal 24 h blood pressure recording showing the diurnal rhythm

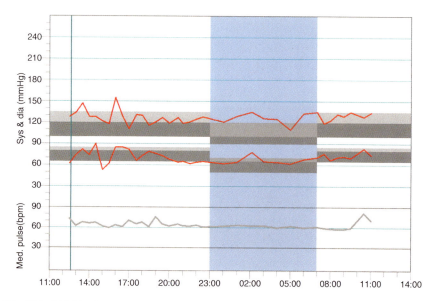

Fig. 10.2   24 h blood pressure recording in someone with chronic kidney disease. Daytime readings are normal but there is no dip during the night

In patients with hypertension, the nocturnal dip may be lost so that the relative elevation in pressure is greater during the night than the day (Fig. 10.3).

The 'white coat' effect tends to be greater in patients with underlying hypertension (Fig. 10.4).

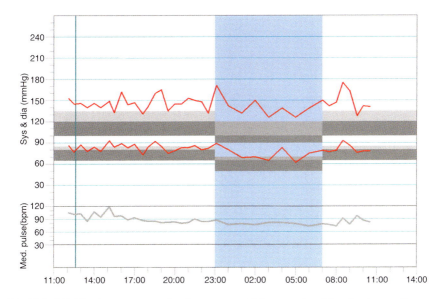

Fig. 10.3 24 h blood pressure recording in someone with hypertension. Most daytime readings are elevated and there is only a small dip during the night. The hypertension is effectively worse during the night

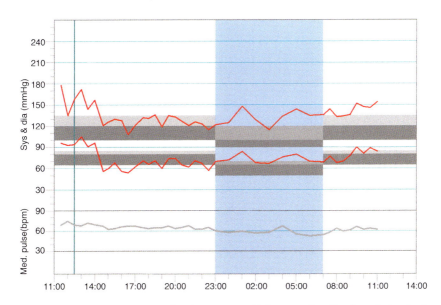

Fig. 10.4 24 h blood pressure recording in someone with hypertension. Readings during the first 3 h are high – the 'white coat' effect. Readings later in the day are normal but there is no dip during the night

In some patients, particularly when chronic kidney disease is more severe, the blood pressure may rise during sleep (Fig 10.5).

The aim of blood pressure treatment should be to restore the normal diurnal variation (Fig. 10.6). Antihypertensive medication taken at night is more likely to

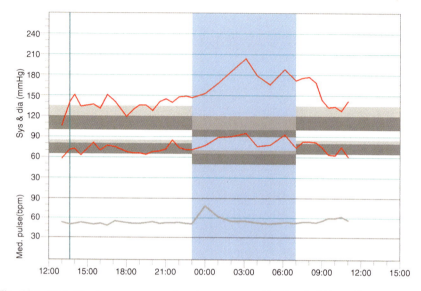

Fig. 10.5 24 h blood pressure recording in someone with chronic kidney disease stage 5, eGFR = 14 ml/min/1.73 m². Readings during the day are nearly normal but during the night they rise dramatically

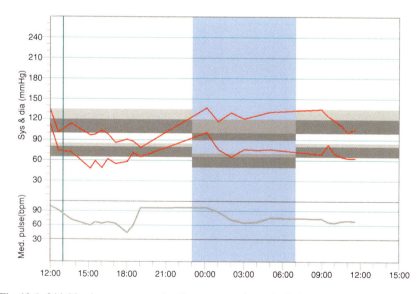

Fig. 10.6 24 h blood pressure recording in someone who took all their blood pressure treatment in the morning. Readings during the day are low after taking the tablets which included a beta blocker – note the drop in pulse rate. The effect of the medication had worn off by the night, leaving the pressure high

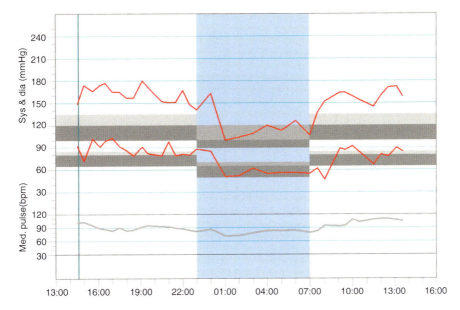

Fig. 10.7 24 h blood pressure recording in someone who took their blood pressure treatment before bedtime. Readings during the night are low after taking the tablets. The daytime pressure was high showing the need for more daytime medication

produce a nocturnal dip (Fig. 10.7) and leads to significantly better cardiovascular outcomes [3]. It can also reduce side effects, such as the swollen ankles caused by calcium channel blockers.

Controlling Blood Pressure – Key to Preserving Kidney Function

Blood pressure control is crucial for slowing the rate of decline in GFR in patients with chronic glomerular disease. The target range should be appropriate for the patient's age. Blood pressure that is low/normal in a young person can cause acute kidney injury in an elderly person who has lost the ability to dilate the kidney arterioles and preserve blood flow when systemic pressure is low – autoregulation (see Sect. "Turning blood into urine" in page 1).

Not all kidney diseases are associated with high blood pressure. Conditions in which the medullary region is damaged, for example ureteric obstruction, can result in the kidneys being unable to conserve sodium. The body is depleted of sodium leading to reduced blood pressure, kidney blood flow and glomerular filtration rate.

In kidney diseases with high blood pressure, lowering the intraglomerular pressure reduces hydrostatic damage to the filtration barrier and slows down glomerulosclerosis. The first sign of this may be a reduction in proteinuria. Inhibitors of the renin-angiotensin-aldosterone system, such as ACE inhibitors and angiotensin receptor blockers (ARBs), are especially effective (see Sect. "ACE inhibitors and angiotensin receptor blockers" in page 104). This is well demonstrated in patients with diabetic nephropathy ("Patient 10.1: Slowing the decline in kidney function with blood pressure control").

Patient 10.1: Slowing the Decline in Kidney Function with Blood Pressure Control

Mr Boss had type 2 diabetes treated with insulin. He had cerebrovascular disease and had undergone coronary artery bypass grafting. He also had ischaemic optic neuropathy and was registered blind.

His blood pressure was poorly controlled; when seen in the diabetes-kidney clinic for the first time in 2008, it was 184/90 mmHg. eGFR had been falling at a rate of 4.5 ml/min/1.73 m^2/year (Fig. 10.8).

His blood pressure treatment was intensified, in particular changing from a thiazide diuretic (indapamide) to a loop diuretic (furosemide) to remove excess salt and water. He learned to measure his blood pressure at home and achieved clinic systolic readings of 125/68 mmHg.

The decline in eGFR slowed to a rate of 1.5 ml/min/1.73 m^2/year (Fig. 10.9).

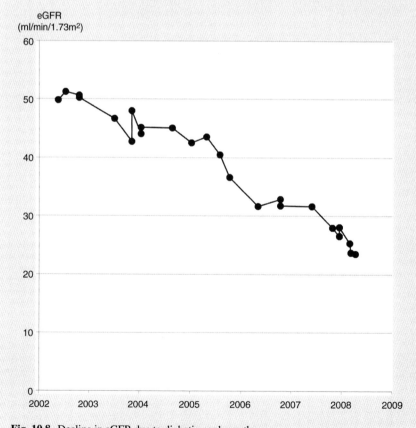

Fig. 10.8 Decline in eGFR due to diabetic nephropathy

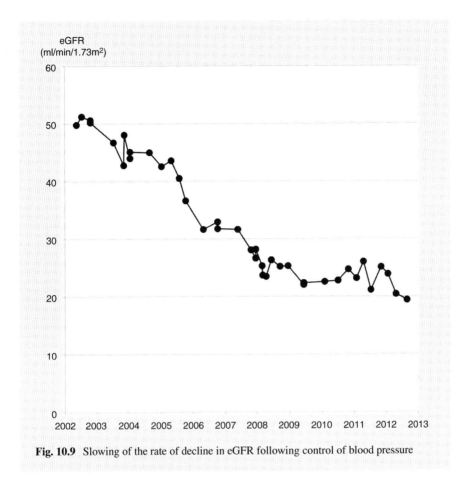

Fig. 10.9 Slowing of the rate of decline in eGFR following control of blood pressure

Controlling blood pressure in patients with malignant hypertension can sometimes reverse the loss of kidney function. The muscular walls of kidney arterioles, which have thickened in reaction to the high pressure, can remodel once the blood pressure is controlled, especially if drugs that inhibit the renin-angiotensin-aldosterone system are used.

References

1. McManus RJ, Mant J, Haque MS, Bray EP, Bryan S, Greenfield SM, Jones MI, Jowett S, Little P, Penaloza C, Schwartz C, Shackleford H, Shovelton C, Varghese J, Williams B, Hobbs FD. Effect of self-monitoring and medication self-titration on systolic blood pressure in hypertensive patients at high risk of cardiovascular disease: the TASMIN-SR randomized clinical trial. JAMA. 2014;312(8):799–808. doi:10.1001/jama.2014.10057. http://jama.jamanetwork.com/article.aspx?articleid=1899205.

2. Clark CE, Aboyans V. Interarm blood pressure difference: more than an epiphenomenon. Nephrol Dial Transplant. 2015;30(5):695–7. doi:10.1093/ndt/gfv075. Epub 2015 Apr 16
3. Hermida RC, Smolensky MH, Ayala DE, Fernández JR, Moyá A, Crespo JJ, Mojón A, Ríos MT, Fabbian F, Portaluppi F. Abnormalities in chronic kidney disease of ambulatory blood pressure 24 h patterning and normalization by bedtime hypertension chronotherapy. Nephrol Dial Transplant. 2013;29(6):1160–7. doi:10.1093/ndt/gft285. http://ndt.oxfordjournals.org/content/early/2013/09/04/ndt.gft285.full.pdf.

Chapter 11
Test the Urine

Understanding Haematuria, Proteinuria and Urinary Infection

Abstract In this chapter we explain:

- How to interpret haematuria
- How myoglobinuria causes acute kidney injury
- The quantification of proteinuria
- Nephrotic syndrome
- How to diagnose urinary infection

Urine testing strips are simple and informative tools for investigating kidney diseases (Fig. 11.1). The assessment of a patient with possible kidney disease is incomplete without urinalysis.

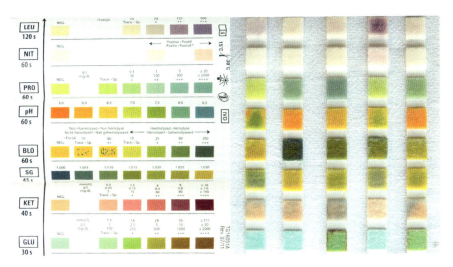

Fig. 11.1 Colour patterns from urine testing strips or 'dipsticks'. The chart on the left is used to interpret the colour changes on the strips on the right

© Springer International Publishing Switzerland 2016
H. Rayner et al., *Understanding Kidney Diseases*,
DOI 10.1007/978-3-319-23458-8_11

Haematuria

Seeing blood in your urine is alarming. As little as 1 mL of blood makes a litre of urine look blood-stained, so the colour exaggerates the amount of blood being lost.

It is important to take a precise history of the appearance of the urine.

• Is it bright red (fresh bleeding) or brick red (altered blood, see Fig. 11.2)?
• Are there clots (urothelial rather than glomerular bleeding)?
• Is the whole stream red from start to finish (blood entered the urine above the bladder outlet)?
• Does the urine start red and then clear (blood from the prostate or urethra washed out by urine from the bladder)?

Men with visible haematuria should have a digital rectal examination and prostate specific antigen serum level measured.

People aged 45 and over with unexplained visible haematuria without urinary tract infection or that persists or recurs after successful treatment of urinary tract infection should be investigated for bladder and kidney cancer. People aged 60 and over with unexplained non-visible haematuria and either dysuria or a raised white cell count on a blood test should similarly be referred [1]. Being on warfarin or other anticoagulant is not an adequate explanation.

The dipstick test distinguishes between free haemoglobin and non-haemolysed red cells (Fig. 11.3). The test strip also reacts to myoglobin. If haemoglobin or myoglobin are released into the circulation they are filtered through the glomeruli and stain the urine dark. Haemoglobinuria occurs with immune-mediated or mechanical

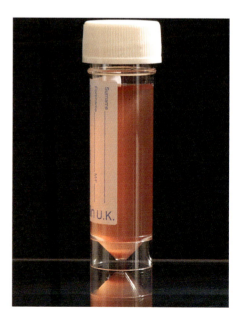

Fig. 11.2 Brick-red urine from a patient with severe acute nephritis. It is opaque due to cells and casts, which form a sediment at the *bottom*

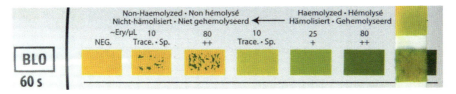

Fig. 11.3 Non-haemolysed microscopic haematuria detected on a urine dipstick test (*right*)

intravascular haemolysis (see Sect. "Kidney disease linked to causes of anaemia" in page 174). Myoglobinuria is discussed in below section "Myoglobinuria".

Dark urine with a negative dipstick test for blood can be caused by food dyes, laxatives containing phenolphthalein, rifampicin and, rarely, by porphyria and alkaptonuria.

How Red Cells Cross the Glomerular Filtration Barrier

If the glomerular filtration barrier is damaged in glomerulonephritis, protein as well as blood can appear in the urine. When combined with reduced GFR and high blood pressure, this constitutes the nephritic syndrome. If the barrier is weakened but otherwise intact, red cells can appear in the urine without protein and with a normal GFR. This is called isolated microscopic haematuria.

Red cells squeeze through the fenestrations in the endothelial cells and cross into Bowman's space. As they pass down the tubule they may become embedded in uromodulin (Tamm-Horsfall protein) and appear in the urine as red cell casts.

Red cells are often damaged as they are forced through the glomerular filtration barrier and so have irregular shapes in the urine. Rarely, they have been caught on electron microscopy in the act of traversing the barrier (Patient 11.1) [2].

Patient 11.1: A Red Cell Caught in the Act

A 22-year-old woman underwent a renal biopsy to investigate persistent microscopic hematuria. There was no macroscopic hematuria, no proteinuria and serum creatinine was normal. There was no family history of kidney disease and no hearing loss.

The glomeruli were normal under light microscopy and immunostaining for immunoglobulins and complement was negative. Electron microscopy showed the capillary walls to be thinner than normal. In one capillary loop, a red blood cell was found almost bisected by the glomerular capillary basement membrane (Fig. 11.4).

Similar pictures of the extravasation of red cells through gaps in endothelial cells have been produced experimentally in frog capillaries exposed to increasing amounts of pressure until they burst [3].

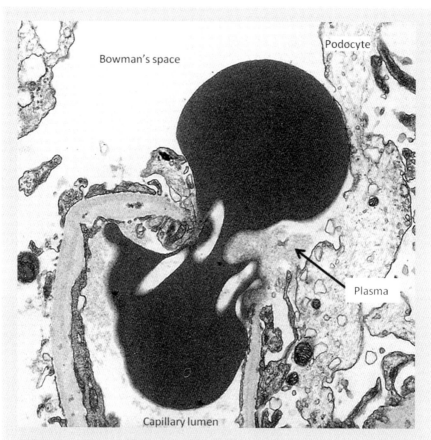

Fig. 11.4 A red cell passing upwards from the capillary lumen at the bottom of the picture through gaps in the cytoplasm of an endothelial cell. The podocyte foot processes have lost contact with the basement membrane and the cell body has been displaced by the red cell. Material similar in density to plasma (*arrow*) is present on the epithelial side of the membrane. This small amount of plasma would have been reabsorbed by the tubule, leaving the red cell alone to appear in the urine (Reproduced with permission from [2])

The Clinical Significance of Haematuria

Although seeing blood in your urine is alarming, haematuria is a less ominous sign than proteinuria in the context of glomerular diseases. For example, thin glomerular basement membrane disease (see Patient 11.1) causes haematuria but is a benign condition that does not lead to kidney failure.

The risk of a fit young person with only microscopic haematuria going on to develop end-stage kidney failure is increased but still very low – 34 versus 2 per 100,000 person years [4].

The commonest type of glomerulonephritis in adults is immunoglobulin A (IgA) nephropathy. It is characterised by the finding in the glomeruli of deposits of IgA. The IgA has abnormally low amounts of galactose bound to it but how this is linked to kidney damage remains unclear. Some patients present with visible (macroscopic) haematuria at the time of a sore throat – synpharyngitic haematuria. (The hematuria in post-streptococcal glomerulonephritis occurs about 2 weeks after the sore throat; see Sect. "Anti-streptolysin O (ASO) and anti-DNAse B antibodies" in page 204) This presentation has a largely benign prognosis, especially when there are repeated episodes of macroscopic haematuria [5].

The risk of kidney failure in patients with IgA nephropathy, and in glomerulonephritis generally, is higher if proteinuria is present, increasing in proportion to the amount of protein. High blood pressure and a reduced eGFR are also signs of a worse prognosis.

The abnormalities on the kidney biopsy in IgA nephropathy can be combined with clinical features to give a prognostic score [6]. Fibrosis in the interstitium is a stronger predictor than many of the glomerular changes. Patients 11.2, 11.3 and 11.4 illustrate the range of outcomes.

Patient 11.2: IgA Nephropathy – Recovery After a Worrying Presentation
Mr. Austin, aged 30 years, presented to hospital with abdominal pain and visible haematuria that had developed after an episode of diarrhoea and vomiting. Urine dipstick showed blood +++ and protein +++. Urine microscopy showed >500 red blood cells/mm^3 but <5 white blood cells/mm^3 and no malignant cells. Culture grew <10^4 organisms/cm^3.

Full blood count was normal and serum creatinine = 86 micromol/L (1 mg/dL). The kidneys looked normal on ultrasound. Plasma immunoglubulins were:

Immunoglobulin IgG	9.98 g/L	(Normal 6.00–16.00)
Immunoglobulin IgA*	3.96 g/L	(0.80–2.80)
Immunoglobulin IgM	1.01 g/L	(0.50–1.90)

*The asterix indicates an abnormal value in the table of results.

Two days after admission, his eGFR dropped to 56 ml/min/1.73 m^2.

A renal biopsy showed 13 largely normal glomeruli but an increase in cells in part of one glomerulus – a segmental glomerulonephritis. Immunofluorescent staining showed many granular deposits of IgA and complement C3 in the mesangial cells of all glomeruli (Fig. 11.5). The mesangial cells lie between the glomerular capillaries and are attached to their basement membrane. They are phagocytic and take up deposits containing IgA and C3 that are trapped by the filtration barrier. These appearances are typical of IgA nephropathy.

Occasional tubules contained red blood cell casts (Fig. 11.6).

The acute kidney injury was attributed to the red cell casts obstructing the tubules [7]. eGFR recovered to its previous level over the following three months (Fig. 11.7).

Three years later Mr. Austin was reviewed in clinic. His urine had been intermittently blood-stained, each time associated with vomiting and joint pain. His serum creatinine was the same as when he first presented – 86 micromol/L (1.0 mg/dL).

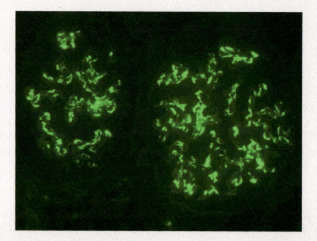

Fig. 11.5 Immunofluorescence microscopy showing positive staining for IgA in the glomerular mesangium. ×400

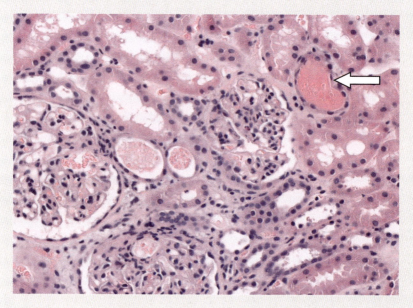

Fig. 11.6 Section through kidney cortex showing glomerular changes of IgA nephropathy, including mesangial hypercellularity and thickening. A number of tubules contain red cell casts, one of which is occluding the lumen (*arrow*). Haematoxylin and eosin ×200

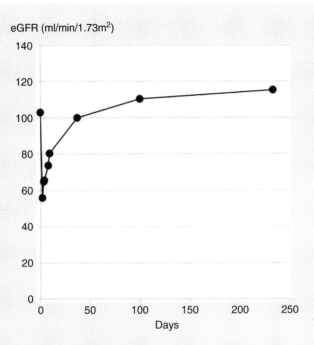

Fig. 11.7 Transient drop in eGFR due to red cell casts in IgA nephropathy

Patient 11.3: IgA Nephropathy – From Haematuria to CKD Stage G5 in 43 Years

Paul first presented in 1971 at the age of 22 years with fever, sore throat, frank haematuria and four episodes of loin pain. His blood pressure was high, ranging from 160/102 to 195/120 mm/Hg. The urine protein/creatinine ratio was 43.1 mg/mmol (380 mg/g) and a 24 h urine collection contained 0.68 g of protein.

A renal biopsy showed some sclerosed glomeruli and others with segmental proliferation consistent with IgA nephropathy. There were some fibrotic scars in the interstitium.

His blood pressure was difficult to control due to drug side effects. However, he remained very fit and twice ran the London marathon in under 4 h.

His kidney function declined over the following 43 years, charted over the last 18 years in Fig. 11.8.

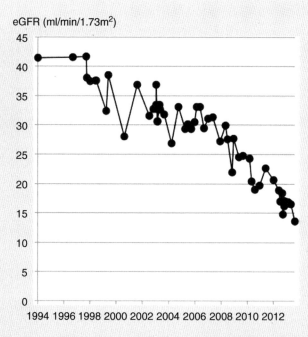

Fig. 11.8 Decline in eGFR at a rate of approximately 2 ml/min/1.73 m²/year due to IgA nephropathy

Patient 11.4: IgA Nephropathy – No Visible Haematuria but End-Stage Kidney Failure in 2 Years

Mr. Mitchell presented for an insurance medical examination at the age of 47. He was a heavy smoker. His urine was found to contain microscopic haematuria and heavy proteinuria, urine protein:creatinine ratio being 565 mg/mmol (4972 mg/g). His eGFR was 69 ml/min/1.73 m².

A renal biopsy specimen showed expansion and increased cellularity of the mesangial region with interstitial and periglomerular fibrosis (Fig. 11.9).

Immunofluorescent staining showed the typical features of IgA nephropathy (Fig. 11.5).

His eGFR rapidly declined over the following 2 years (Fig. 11.10). Smoking may have accelerated the decline; smokers with IgA nephropathy are twice as likely to lose kidney function [8].

He later had a successful kidney transplant.

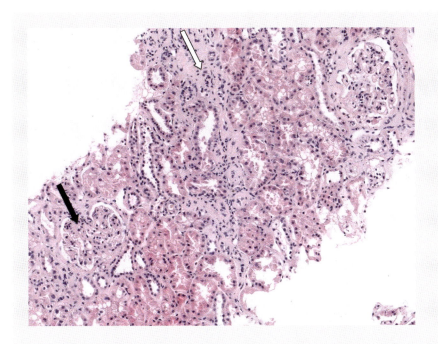

Fig. 11.9 Light micrograph showing expansion and hypercellularity of the mesangial region with glomerulosclerosis (*black arrow*). There is interstitial fibrosis and tubular atrophy, best seen as a vertical band of pale cellular tissue between the tubules in the middle of the section (*white arrow*) and around the glomerulus in the upper right corner. Haematoxylin and eosin ×100

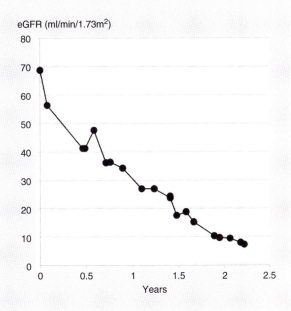

Fig. 11.10 Decline in eGFR at a rate of 30 ml/min/1.73 m^2/year due to IgA nephropathy

Myoglobinuria

Myoglobinuria results from the breakdown of large amounts of muscle tissue. Physical damage can be due to compression from prolonged immobility or crush injury, ischaemia from embolism, electric shock or severe exercise induced by recreational drugs (Patient 11.5). Prescribed drugs, notably statins, and infectious or inflammatory diseases that cause myositis can cause muscle breakdown. Metabolic conditions such as McArdle disease, hypokalaemia or an enzyme deficiency make the muscles vulnerable to damage [9].

A number of mechanisms lead to acute kidney injury with myoglobinuria. Necrotic muscle swells up leading to hypovolaemia and shock. Myoglobin is concentrated in the tubules where it precipitates with uromodulin to form casts that obstruct the flow of filtrate. Increased uric acid production from muscle protein leads to uric acid casts, which are more likely to precipitate in the low urine pH caused by metabolic acidosis. And finally, the haem centre of the molecule is toxic to the tubular cells which reabsorb the filtered myoglobin.

The exposed sarcoplasm and myofibrils in damaged muscle release potassium and phosphate into the circulation and bind calcium, causing hypocalcaemia and cardiac arrhythmias. The damaged muscles can become calcified. The bound calcium is released during the recovery phase as the muscles heal, causing hypercalcaemia.

Patient 11.5: Rhabdomyolyisis, Myoglobinuria and Acute Kidney Injury
Ryan, a 23-year-old unemployed man, was admitted as an emergency having been found unconscious on the floor. He had lain there for at least 12 h. He had a history of epilepsy and alcohol dependency, and used intravenous heroin.

On arrival at the casualty department, the skin over his legs had already begun to blister from pressure damage, and his muscles were tense. He was oliguric and his urine was like cola (Fig. 11.11).

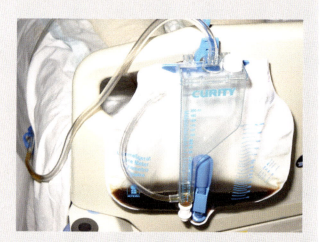

Fig. 11.11 Cola-coloured urine due to myoglobinuria

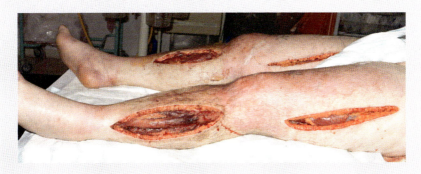

Fig. 11.12 Multiple fasciotomies revealing necrotic muscle. There is blistering of the skin by the right knee caused by prolonged pressure and oedema

His serum creatinine had increased from 78 micromols/L (0.9 mg/dL) seven months previously to 172 (1.9) on arrival and 297 (3.4) 13 h later (stage 3 AKI; see Table 3.2). Serum creatine phosphokinase was >50,000 IU/L.

On arrival, his serum potassium was high (8.6 mmol/L, mEq/L) and calcium low (corrected for serum albumin = 1.78 mmol/L, 7.1 mg/dL) due to the release of potassium and binding of calcium by damaged muscle fibres.

Because the pressure within all the muscle compartments of his legs was extremely high, 100–125 mmHg, multiple fasciotomies were performed. The muscles were swollen and some visibly necrotic (Fig. 11.12).

Proteinuria

Normal glomerular filtration allows an estimated 3.3–5.7 g of albumin per day to pass into the proximal tubule. This is almost all reabsorbed and very little appears in the urine. If the filtration barrier is damaged, the amount of albumin and other proteins that pass into the tubule can overwhelm its absorptive capacity so that much more appears in the urine (Fig. 11.13).

Large amounts of albumin make the urine foamy. Normal urine can make froth if it is concentrated and rapidly urinated or if it contains large amount of semen due to retrograde ejaculation. Bubbly urine can be passed in patients with a vesicocolic fistula or infection with gas forming organisms.

Perhaps surprisingly, the passage of albumin across the filtration barrier is easier when the thickness of the glomerular basement membrane is increased (Fig. 11.14). Conversely, patients with thin basement membranes do not have proteinuria (see Sect. "How red cells cross the glomerular filtration barrier" in page 135). It is the structural integrity and the size and electrical charge of pores in the membrane rather than its thickness that determine how easily proteins can pass through.

Testing for and quantifying albuminuria or proteinuria are an essential part of the assessment of someone with kidney disease. The amount of albumin lost per day is most easily measured by calculating the ratio of the concentration of albumin to the concentration of creatinine in a sample of urine:

Fig. 11.13 Heavy proteinuria on a urine dipstick test (*PRO +++*)

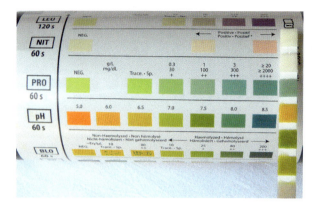

Fig. 11.14 Electron micrograph showing thickening of the glomerular basement membrane up to 786 nm in a patient with diabetes and nephrotic range proteinuria. The average width of a normal glomerular basement membrane is 280 nm. Magnification 9300×

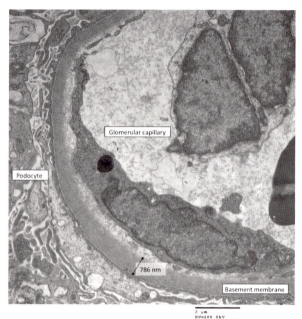

$$\text{Albumin:creatinine ratio (ACR)} = \frac{\text{Urine albumin concentration}}{\text{Urine creatinine concentration}}$$

The protein:creatinine ratio (PCR) is calculated in a similar way.

Using the ratio removes the effect of changes in the dilution of urine from hour to hour and day to day. If the urine is more dilute, the concentrations of both albumin and creatinine are reduced and so the ratio remains the same. As the rate of production of creatinine remains fairly constant from day to day, sequential ACR results show the trend in the rate of albuminuria.

Table 11.1 Stages of albuminuria

A1: normal – male	ACR <2.5 mg/mmol	<20 mg/g
A1: normal – female	ACR <3.5 mg/mmol	<30 mg/g
A2: microalbuminuria – male	ACR 2.5–30 mg/mmol	20 to <300 mg/g
A2: microalbuminuria – female	ACR 3.5–30 mg/mmol	30 to <300 mg/g
A3: macroalbuminuria	ACR >30 mg/mmol	>300 mg/g
Nephrotic-range proteinuria [10]	ACR >220 mg/mmol	>2200 mg/g
	PCR >350 mg/mmol	>3500 mg/g

In UK laboratories, ACR and PCR are reported as mg protein per mmol creatinine. Although the daily excretion rate of creatinine varies according to muscle mass, a convenient average figure is 10 mmol creatinine per day. Multiplying the ACR or PCR in mg/mmol by ten gives an estimate of the number of grams of protein lost per day.

In the US, ACR and PCR are expressed as mg/g. This is 8.8 times the value in mg/mmol and is similar to the amount in milligrams per day in a 24 h urine collection.

Table 11.1 shows the conventional stages of albuminuria in mg/mmol, with their equivalents in mg/g.

Chronic kidney disease is staged according to the eGFR and the ACR. For example, a man with CKD stage G4A2 would have an eGFR 15–29 ml/min/1.73 m^2 and an albumin:creatinine ratio 2.5–30 mg/mmol.

Figure 11.15 compares albuminuria and proteinuria in a patient with diabetes. 30 mg/mmol (250 mg/g) of albuminuria, the threshold between microalbuminuria and proteinuria, is equivalent to 45 mg/mmol (400 mg/g) of proteinuria. The difference is predominantly made up of uromodulin (Tamm-Horsfall protein) secreted by the distal tubules (see Sect. "Uromodulin" in page 90).

It is best to use the first sample of urine passed in the day to measure the ACR. Losses of albumin increase with exercise, blood pressure and salt intake, and so are higher and more variable during the day than during the night. There is considerable variation in ACR on a morning sample from day to day. In someone with an ACR >30 mg/mmol, a difference of more than 83 % between two samples is needed to be confident that there has been a real change in the underlying disease [11].

The long-term trend in ACR or PCR is a useful guide to changes in kidney disease. A progressive and sustained reduction in proteinuria is an encouraging sign that treatment, such as improved control of blood pressure, is working. The opposite trend highlights the need for better control (Fig. 11.16).

Whether proteinuria actually damages nephrons and so contributes directly to the progression of disease has been the subject of much debate. If it does, reducing proteinuria would in itself be a worthy aim. Proteinuria has been used as a surrogate endpoint for many trials investigating whether drugs slow the progression of CKD. Changes in proteinuria can be measured over a shorter timescale than changes in mortality, so we get a quicker answer [12].

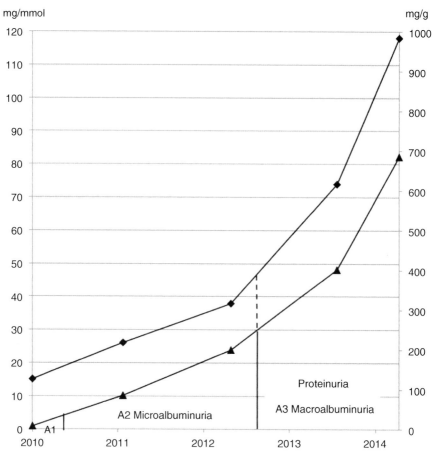

Fig. 11.15 Simultaneous measurements of urinary protein:creatinine ratio (*upper line*) and albumin:creatinine ratio (*lower line*) in a patient with increasing proteinuria due to diabetic nephropathy

But changes in proteinuria may not be a reliable guide to hard endpoints. For example, giving patients with diabetic nephropathy a combination of two drugs that inhibit the renin-angiotensin-aldosterone system may lead to a reduction in proteinuria and a slowing of the rate of decline in eGFR over the short term. Unfortunately, with longer follow-up it is clear that they may also cause acute kidney injury and do not reduce the risk of mortality or cardiovascular events [13].

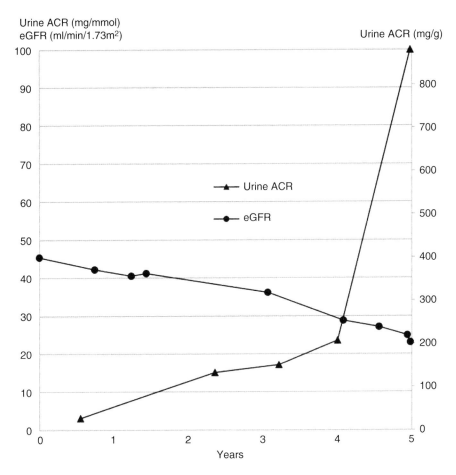

Fig. 11.16 Trends in urine albumin:creatinine ratio and eGFR in a man with diabetic nephropathy showing a progressive increase in albuminuria and reduction in glomerular filtration rate

Patient 11.6: The Effect of a Combination of ACEI and ARB
Robert was treated for his diabetic nephropathy with the ACE-inhibitor lisino-pril for many years. Because his blood pressure remained too high and eGFR was falling, the angiotensin receptor blocker (ARB) irbesartan was added in 2003 (Fig. 11.17).

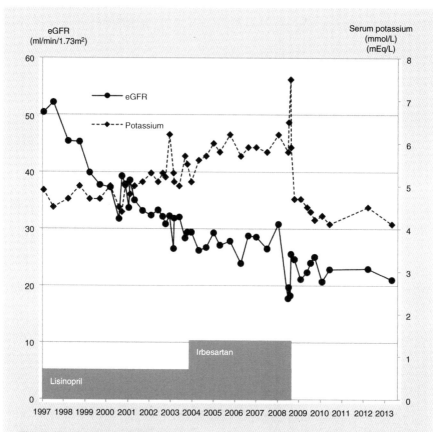

Fig. 11.17 Changes in eGFR and serum potassium in a patient with diabetic nephropathy treated with initially an ACE inhibitor and then combined with an angiotensin receptor blocker

In 2006 a systematic review of this combination [14] concluded "the combination of ACE-inhibitor and ARB therapy … is safe, without clinically meaningful changes in serum potassium levels or glomerular filtration rates (and) a significant decrease in proteinuria … in the short term".

Over the next 4 years his eGFR remained stable and his serum potassium was elevated but safe. But in 2008, without any warning, there was sudden drop in eGFR, and a rise in urea to 22 mmol/L (BUN=62 mg/dL) and potassium to 7.5 mmol/L (mEq/L).

Both lisinopril and irbesartan were stopped, serum potassium returned to normal and there was an improvement in eGFR, although not back to the previous level. From showing no proteinuria, his urine dipstick now showed +++ protein. Thereafter, despite the recurrence of proteinuria, the eGFR remained stable, raising doubts about the apparent benefit of the drug combination seen from 2004.

This patient encapsulates the results of the VA-NEPHRON D study and other studies, which have led to a European Union recommendation not to prescribe an ACE inhibitor and angiotensin receptor blocker together.

Nephrotic Syndrome

When the rate of loss of albumin into the urine exceeds the rate of albumin synthesis by the liver, the concentration of albumin in the serum starts to fall. It is like trying to keep up the level of water in a bath when the plug is leaking. Turning the tap on fully will initially keep the level up but if the leak gets worse the level will start to drop.

The amount of albumin synthesized by the liver per day is normally about 0.1 g/kg body weight, i.e. 7 g for an average 70 kg person [15]. This is increased in the nephrotic syndrome but so too is the rate of breakdown of albumin. When albuminuria exceeds 3.5 g per 1.73 m^2 of body-surface area per day, i.e. 5 g for an average adult, liver synthesis cannot keep up and serum albumin falls.

The increase in protein synthesis also affects the production of apolipoproteins by the liver. As a result, patients with nephrotic syndrome usually have high serum cholesterol levels, often over 10 mmol/L (400 mg/dL).

Nephrotic syndrome is a triad of urine albumin excretion >3.5 g per 1.73 m^2 per day, serum albumin concentration $\leq$25 g/L ($\leq$2.5 g/dL) and oedema (Fig. 11.18). Rather than analysing a full 24 h collection, the albuminuria is more easily estimated from the urine protein:creatinine ratio, nephrotic range being above 350 mg/mmol (3500 mg/g) in adults and 200 mg/mmol (2000 mg/g) in children.

All three criteria must be met to make a diagnosis of nephrotic syndrome. Low serum albumin and oedema without albuminuria can be found in many conditions. For example, chronic liver disease causes oedema due to salt retention and low serum albumin due to reduced synthesis. Systemic inflammation reduces serum albumin by depressing its rate of synthesis and increasing its breakdown. For this reason, serum albumin is described as a negative acute-phase reactant.

The oedema in nephrotic syndrome is commonly put down to reduced oncotic pressure from the low serum albumin allowing salt and water to leak into the tissues. However, this traditional explanation is not the full story [16]. For example, adults with congenital analbuminaemia, an autosomal recessive disorder where serum albumin is absent, have a low plasma oncotic pressure but little or no oedema.

The oedema of nephrotic syndrome is actually caused by retention of sodium by the kidneys combined with increased permeability of the capillary walls allowing fluid to leak into the tissues. Children with nephrotic syndrome that responds to steroid treatment excrete the excess sodium as soon as the proteinuria stops and before the serum albumin recovers.

Because the tubules are reabsorbing sodium along much of the length of the nephron, diuretics given at usual doses are often ineffective in nephrotic syndrome. Much higher doses of loop diuretics, sometimes in combination with a thiazide diuretic, are needed to block sodium reabsorption along a sufficient length of the nephron to achieve a diuresis (see Fig. 7.3).

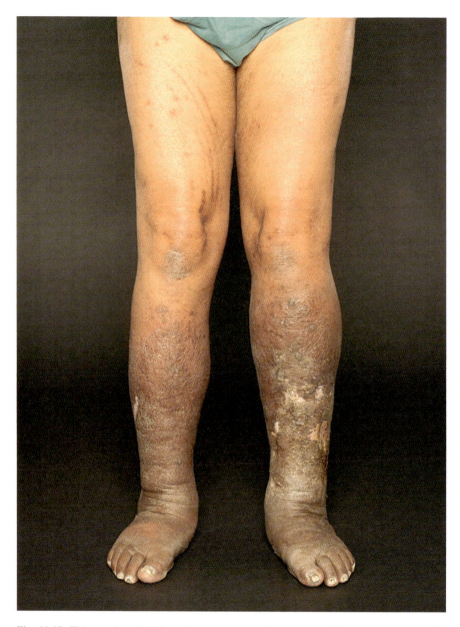

Fig. 11.18 This man has chronic nephrotic syndrome due to severe diabetic nephropathy. The urine protein:creatinine ratio was 549 mg/mmol (4831 mg/g) and the serum albumin was 19 g/L (1.9 g/dL). The oedema in his legs has caused pigmented thickening (lichenification) of the skin and ulceration. The ulcers have healed leaving white scars

A renal biopsy is often performed to identify the pathological features of the nephrotic syndrome. An abnormality in all patients is fusion of the podocyte foot processes (Fig. 11.19). The digits of the podocyte merge across the slit diaphragm

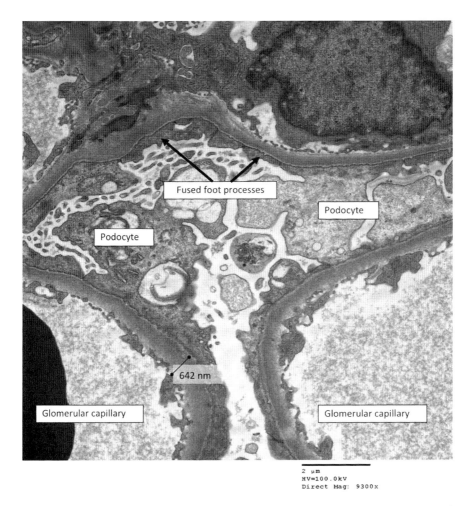

Fused foot processes

Podocyte

Podocyte

642 nm

Glomerular capillary   Glomerular capillary

2 μm
HV=100.0kV
Direct Mag: 9300x

Fig. 11.19 Electron micrograph showing complete fusion of the podocyte foot processes and thickening of the glomerular basement membrane in a patient with minimal change nephrotic syndrome. The average width of a normal membrane is 280 nm. Magnification 9300×

to form a continuous layer over the surface of the glomerular basement membrane. The width of the basement membrane is increased, suggesting that the collagen protein molecules are packed less tightly together, allowing protein molecules to pass between them. These changes are only visible under the electron microscope. Under light microscopy the specimen may show no definite abnormalities, in which case it is called minimal change nephrotic syndrome.

Acute kidney injury may sometimes accompany the onset of nephrotic syndrome. This is more often due to changes in the glomerular filtration barrier and podocyte foot process fusion rather than plasma volume reduction and reduced renal blood flow [17].

Patients with nephrotic syndrome are at risk of venous thrombosis due to the loss of antithrombin III in the urine. Antithrombin III is an anticoagulant protein that has a molecular weight lower than serum albumin (58.2 kDa compared to 66.5 kDa). Clotting can occur in unusual venous territories such as the renal, cerebral or mesenteric veins [18]. The lower the serum albumin, the greater is the risk. A serum albumin <20 g/l (<2 g/dL) is a useful rule of thumb for considering prophylactic anticoagulation, and more sophisticated predictive tools have been developed [19].

Immunoglobulins and complement are also lost into the urine, increasing the risk of infections, particularly in children and in developing countries [20].

Urine Infection

Infection in the urinary tract presents with a range of symptoms and signs (Fig. 11.20). This section explains an approach to diagnosing infection and its cause.

Figure 11.21 shows a dipstick urine test from Adele, a teenage girl with bilateral vesicoureteric reflux and scarring of both kidneys. She has had recurrent attacks of burning dysuria and loin pain. Does she have a urine infection?

In a woman, the best guide to whether a urine infection is present are her symptoms - frequency, dysuria, haematuria, fever, loin pain – and the absence of vaginal irritation or discharge. If the symptoms are present when the urine is tested, the dipstick test does not add much; whatever the stick test shows, a urine culture is needed.

The stick tests for nitrites and leucocytes are best used as 'rule-out' tests. A negative urine dipstick test for both nitrites and leucocytes makes a UTI unlikely, but an MSU culture should still be done in patients with symptoms. If someone has only loin pain and a negative urine dipstick test for nitrites and leucocytes, urinary infection is unlikely to be the cause of the pain [21].

Although Adele's urine is ++ for leucocytes and positive for nitrites, she had no symptoms at the time of the sample and her urine culture was negative. She did not have sufficient evidence to warrant antibiotic treatment at that time but is at high risk of future infection because of her reflux nephropathy.

Urine infection most certainly cannot be diagnosed from a positive urine dipstick test for blood and/or protein. Despite this, a very high proportion of older people presenting to a doctor with blood and protein on a urine dipstick test are given a diagnosis of '?UTI' and inappropriately started on antibiotics.

As urine flows out of the urethra is can be contaminated by organisms from the skin surface. The number of organisms (Colony Forming Units) grown from a correctly collected MSU specimen that distinguishes between contaminants and an infection is >10^5 CFU/ml. A diagnosis of UTI can be made in a patient with a colony count above this threshold *and* symptoms suggestive of infection.

The presence of symptoms is crucial for interpreting an MSU culture result. Many older women, especially with diabetes, yield a significant growth but have no symptoms. They are colonised with organisms and treatment with antibiotics does not lead to improved kidney function or a lower risk of future symptomatic urine infections. Treatment of asymptomatic bacteriuria is only indicated in pregnant women or prior to invasive urological surgery [22].

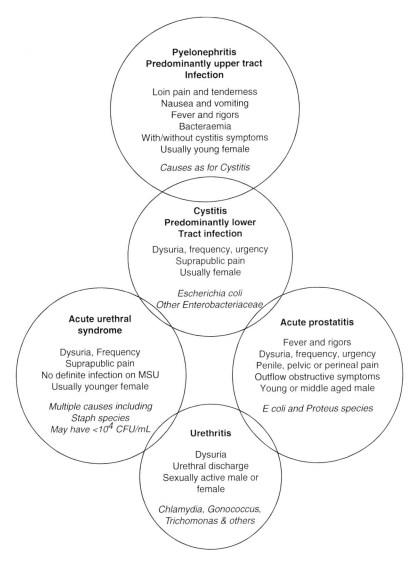

Fig. 11.20 Acute urinary tract infection syndromes in adults. Although shown as discrete syndromes they may overlap. The commoner causative organisms are in *italics*

Dipstick tests on urine specimens taken from a urinary catheter (CSU) are even less meaningful than an MSU. The culture result can be interpreted as for an MSU. A positive culture without systemic symptoms does not warrant treatment with antibiotics because the catheter is likely to be coated with a biofilm containing the micro-organisms. The risk of colonisation of the catheter increases by about 5 % per day after insertion.

Specimens from a nephrostomy should be highlighted to the laboratory. The sample is less likely to be contaminated so all organisms will be separately identified to guide antimicrobial treatment.

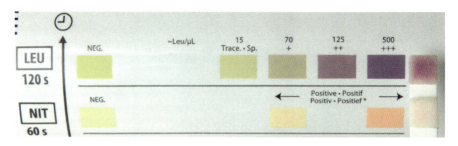

Fig. 11.21 Leucocytes and nitrites detected on a urine dipstick test

People aged 60 and over with recurrent or persistent unexplained urinary tract infection should be considered for investigation for bladder cancer [1].

It is important to take a sexual history in all women with a UTI. The likelihood of urine infection in both pre- and post- menopausal women is associated with the frequency of sexual intercourse [23, 24].

In men, urine infection is much less common and should always prompt a search for an underlying cause. The species of organism grown may give a clue. For example, *Proteus mirabilis* produce urease, which breaks down urea and reduces the acidity of urine, leading to the formation of kidney or bladder stones. The bacteria then stick to the stone where they are protected from antibiotics.

Infection that ascends into the kidney – pyelonephritis – causes loin pain and high fever. It rarely affects the GFR because the infection does not obstruct the tubules. If the eGFR is reduced, a structural cause should be looked for, especially if a more unusual organism is grown (Patient 11.7).

Patient 11.7: Unusual Urinary Infection Suggests an Underlying Pathology

Angie, aged 36, presented to her GP with symptoms of a urine infection. She had had urinary frequency and pain on and off over the previous ten months. A mid-stream urine sample subsequently yielded a heavy growth of *Enterococcus faecalis* and she was treated with antibiotics according to the organism's sensitivities. The GP also measured her renal function and the eGFR was only 17 ml/min/1.73 m^2. She was sent urgently to hospital.

In the emergency assessment unit, she described having left lower back pain for the previous 2 days. She had intense urinary frequency, having to go to the toilet halfway through the conversation.

An ultrasound scan of the kidneys and bladder showed bilateral hydronephrosis, with marked thinning of the renal cortex on the right indicating chronic damage. The left kidney cortex was thicker suggesting more recent obstruction, consistent with her symptoms (Fig. 11.22).

In the pelvis there was a central solid mass adherent to the bladder. When asked about any previous gynaecological problems, she said she had had a hysterectomy for cervical carcinoma 5 years previously.

By this time, her eGFR had dropped to 7 ml/min/1.73 m^2. Bilateral neph-rostomies were inserted (Fig. 11.23) and her kidney function improved over the next 10 days (Fig. 11.24).

An MRI scan confirmed the ultrasound scan findings (Fig. 11.25).

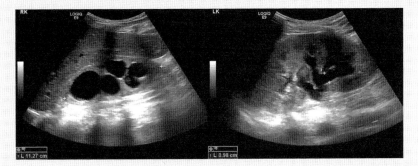

Fig. 11.22 Ultrasound scan showing bilateral hydronephrosis, with marked thinning of the right renal cortex (*RK right kidney, LK left kidney*)

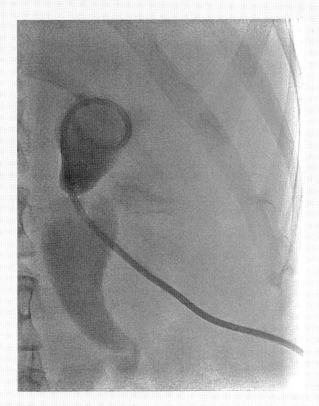

Fig. 11.23 Nephrostogram showing hydronephrosis and a dilated upper ureter

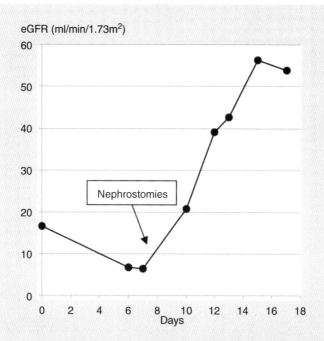

Fig. 11.24 Relief of obstruction by nephrostomies led to recovery in kidney function

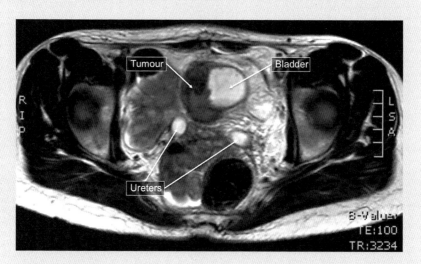

Fig. 11.25 MRI scan on the pelvis showing a tumour adjacent to the bladder and dilated ureters

A nuclear medicine whole body fluoro-deoxyglucose Positron Emission Tomography scan (FDG PET scan) (Fig. 11.26) combined with CT (Fig 11.27) showed marked activity in the mass adjacent to the bladder, consistent with recurrent cervical carcinoma.

The nephrostomies were replaced by bilateral ureteric stents and she was transferred to the oncology unit for a course of chemotherapy and radiotherapy.

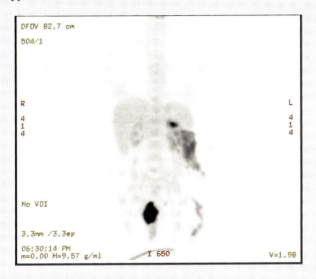

Fig. 11.26 FDG PET scan showing high level of activity in the pelvis

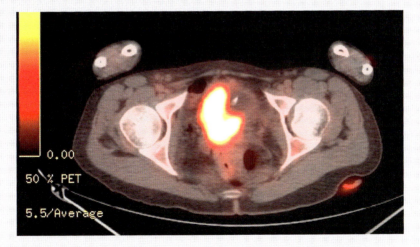

Fig. 11.27 PET CT scan showing that the high level of radioactivity is located in the tumour mass

References

1. National Collaborating Centre for Cancer. Suspected cancer: recognition and referral. NICE Guideline. 2015. http://www.nice.org.uk/guidance/NG12/chapter/1-recommendations#urological-cancers.
2. Collar JE, Ladva S, Cairns TDH, Cattell V. Red cell traverse through thin glomerular basement membranes. Kidney Int. 2001;59:2069–72. doi:10.1046/j.1523-1755.2001.00721.x. http://www.nature.com/ki/journal/v59/n6/full/4492253a.html#bib7.
3. Neal CR, Michel CC. Openings in frog microvascular endothelium induced by high intravascular pressures. J Physiol. 1996;492(1):39–52.
4. Vivante A, Afek A, Frenkel-Nir Y, Tzur D, Farfel A, Golan E, Chaiter Y, Shohat T, Skorecki K, Calderon-Margalit R. Persistent asymptomatic isolated microscopic hematuria in Israeli adolescents and young adults and risk for end-stage renal disease. JAMA. 2011;306(7):729–36. doi:10.1001/jama.2011.1141. http://jama.jamanetwork.com/article.aspx?articleid=1104231.
5. Le W, Liang S, Chen H, Wang S, Zhang W, Wang X, Wang J, Zeng C-H, Liu Z-H. Long-term outcome of IgA nephropathy patients with recurrent macroscopic hematuria. Am J Nephrol. 2014;40:43–50. http://www.karger.com/Article/Abstract/364954.
6. Roberts IS. Oxford classification of immunoglobulin A nephropathy: an update. Curr Opin Nephrol Hypertens. 2013;22(3):281–6. doi:10.1097/MNH.0b013e32835fe65c. http://journals.lww.com/co-nephrolhypertens/Abstract/2013/05000/Oxford_classification_of_immunoglobulin_A.6.aspx.
7. Gutiérrez E, González E, Hernández E, Morales E, Martínez MA, Usera G, Praga M. Factors that determine an incomplete recovery of renal function in macrohematuria-induced acute renal failure of IgA nephropathy. Clin J Am Soc Nephrol. 2007;2(1):51. http://cjasn.asnjournals.org/content/2/1/51.long.
8. Yamamoto R, Nagasawa Y, Shoji T, Iwatani H, Hamano T, Kawada N, Inoue K, Uehata T, Kaneko T, Okada N, Moriyama T, Horio M, Yamauchi A, Tsubakihara Y, Imai E, Rakugi H, Isaka Y. Cigarette smoking and progression of IgA nephropathy. Am J Kidney Dis. 2010;56(2):313. http://www.ajkd.org/article/S0272-6386(10)00682-7/abstract.
9. Vanholder R, Sever MS, Erek E, Lameire N. Rhabdomyolysis. J Am Soc Nephrol. 2000;11:1553–61. http://jasn.asnjournals.org/content/11/8/1553.full.
10. Stoycheff N, Stevens LA, Schmid CH, Tighiouart H, Lewis J, Atkins RC, Levey AS. Nephrotic syndrome in diabetic kidney disease: an evaluation and update of the definition. Am J Kidney Dis. 2009;54(5):840–9. doi:10.1053/j.ajkd.2009.04.016. Epub 2009 Jun 25. http://www.ncbi.nlm.nih.gov/pmc/articles/PMC4036614/.
11. Naresh CN, Hayen A, Weening A, Craig JC, Chadban SJ. Day-to-day variability in spot urine albumin-creatinine ratio. Am J Kidney Dis. 2013;62(6):1095–101. http://www.ajkd.org/article/S0272-6386(13)01007-X/abstract.
12. Lambers Heerspink HJ, Kröpelin TF, Hoekman J, Zeeuw D, on behalf of the Reducing Albuminuria as Surrogate Endpoint (REASSURE) Consortium. Drug-induced reduction in albuminuria is associated with subsequent renoprotection: a meta-analysis. J Am Soc Nephrol. doi:10.1681/ASN.2014070688. http://jasn.asnjournals.org/content/early/2014/11/23/ASN.2014070688.abstract.
13. Fried LF, Emanuele N, Zhang JH, Brophy M, Conner TA, Duckworth W, Leehey DJ, McCullough PA, O'Connor T, Palevsky PM, Reilly RF, Seliger SL, Warren SR, Watnick S, Peduzzi P, Guarino P, VA NEPHRON-D Investigators. Combined angiotensin inhibition for the treatment of diabetic nephropathy. N Engl J Med. 2013;369(20):1892–903. doi:10.1056/NEJMoa1303154. Epub 2013 Nov 9. http://www.nejm.org/doi/full/10.1056/NEJMoa1303154#t=articleTop.
14. MacKinnon M, Shurraw S, Akbari A, Knoll GA, Jaffey J, Clark HD. Combination therapy with an angiotensin receptor blocker and an ACE inhibitor in proteinuric renal disease: a systematic review of the efficacy and safety data. Am J Kidney Dis. 2006;48(1):8–20. http://www.ajkd.org/article/S0272-6386(06)00769-4/abstract.

15. Barle H, Nyberg B, Essén P, Andersson K, McNurlan MA, Wernerman J, Garlick PJ. The synthe- sis rates of total liver protein and plasma albumin determined simultaneously in vivo in humans. Hepatology. 1997;25(1):154–8. http://onlinelibrary.wiley.com/doi/10.1002/hep.510250128/epdf.
16. Doucet A, Favre G, Deschênes G. Molecular mechanism of edema formation in nephrotic syndrome: therapeutic implications. Pediatr Nephrol. 2007;22:1983–90. doi:10.1007/ s00467-007-0521-3. http://www.ncbi.nlm.nih.gov/pmc/articles/PMC2064946/.
17. Smith JD, Hayslett JP. Reversible renal failure in the nephrotic syndrome. Am J Kidney Dis. 1992;19(3):201.
18. Loscalzo J. Venous thrombosis in the nephrotic syndrome. N Engl J Med. 2013;368:956–8. doi:10.1056/NEJMcibr1209459. http://www.nejm.org/doi/full/10.1056/NEJMcibr1209459.
19. Lee T, Biddle AK, Lionaki S, Derebail VK, Barbour SJ, Tannous S, Hladunewich MA, Hu Y, Poulton CJ, Mahoney SL, Jennette JC, Hogan SL, Falk RL, Cattran DC, Reich HN, Nachman PH. Personalized prophylactic anticoagulation decision analysis in patients with membranous nephropathy. Kidney Int. 2014;85(6):1412–20. doi:10.1038/ki.2013.476. http://www.nature. com/ki/journal/v85/n6/full/ki2013476a.html.
20. Alwadhi RK, Mathew JL, Rath B. Clinical profile of children with nephrotic syndrome not on glucocorticoid therapy, but presenting with infection. J Paediatr Child Health. 2004;40(1–2):28– 32. http://onlinelibrary.wiley.com/doi/10.1111/j.1440-1754.2004.00285.x/abstract.
21. St John A, Boyd JC, Lowes AJ, Price CP. The use of urinary dipstick tests to exclude urinary tract infection: a systematic review of the literature. Am J Clin Pathol. 2006;126(3):428–36. http://ajcp.ascpjournals.org/content/126/3/428.full.pdf.
22. Nicolle LE, Bradley S, Colgan R, Rice JC, Schaeffer A, Hooton TM, Infectious Diseases Society of America; American Society of Nephrology; American Geriatric Society. Infectious Diseases Society of America guidelines for the diagnosis and treatment of asymptomatic bac- teriuria in adults. Clin Infect Dis. 2005;40(5):643–54. Epub 2005 Feb 4. http://www.idsociety. org/uploadedFiles/IDSA/Guidelines-Patient_Care/PDF_Library/Asymptomatic%20 Bacteriuria.pdf.
23. Hooton TM, Scholes D, Hughes JP, Winter C, Roberts PL, Stapleton AE, Stergachis A, Stamm WE. A prospective study of risk factors for symptomatic urinary tract infection in young women. N Engl J Med. 1996;335(7):468–74. http://www.nejm.org/doi/full/10.1056/NEJM19 9608153350703#t=articleTop.
24. Moore EE, Hawes SE, Scholes D, Boyko EJ, Hughes JP, Fihn SD. Sexual intercourse and risk of symptomatic urinary tract infection in post-menopausal women. J Gen Intern Med. 2008;23(5):595–9. doi:10.1007/s11606-008-0535-y. Epub 2008 Feb 12. http://link.springer. com/article/10.1007%2Fs11606-008-0535-y.

Chapter 12
Examine the Patient

Physical Signs Related to Kidney Diseases

Abstract In this chapter we explain:

- How to assess fluid balance
- The importance of examining the abdomen
- Common signs of a vasculitic illness

This chapter is placed after the chapters on history, height, weight, blood pressure and urine testing because the physical examination should be tailored according to these results. The blood pressure and urinalysis may have been tested before you see the patient. If not, include them as part of your examination.

Fluid Balance

How Salt and Water Is Distributed in the Body

Salt and water are distributed in three functionally separate compartments – inside the cells (intracellular fluid), around the cells (interstitial fluid) and in blood vessels (plasma).

Before trying to judge a patient's salt and water balance from the physical examination, first take a history. For example, if someone has had diarrhoea and vomiting for a week and has lost weight they will be salt and water depleted. The examination is then used to judge the severity of the salt and water depletion and whether it is affecting plasma volume as well as interstitial fluid.

In children, the percentage change in body weight is used to guide the route and volume of fluid replacement. Weight loss of more than 10 % of body weight indicates reduced plasma volume and requires intravenous fluid replacement. In adults, low blood pressure and a rise in pulse rate of >20 bpm from sitting to standing or >30 bpm from supine to standing indicate reduced plasma volume.

Traditional signs of reduced interstitial fluid volume such as reduced skin turgor are not reliable in the elderly [1].

Oedema indicates excess interstitial fluid. Interstitial fluid is formed at the arterial end of the capillary bed by hydrostatic pressure forcing fluid across the capillary wall. It is removed at the venous end by osmotic force drawing it back into the capillary lumen, and also by the lymphatic system (Fig. 12.1).

Salt and water overload leads to increased hydrostatic pressure and oedema. A little puffiness at the ankles indicates a kilogram or two of excess fluid. Oedema to the knees may indicate five kilograms; oedema up to the abdomen may mean more than 20 kg of fluid overload. Fluid may also accumulate in spaces that are normally dry, for example as pleural effusions and ascites.

Older people develop oedema more readily than younger people. It can be hard to detect fluid overload in younger patients as they become hypertensive but do not show oedema. Patients with low serum albumin tend to form oedema more easily due to the reduced capillary osmotic pressure.

Interstitial fluid can flow within subcutaneous tissue. This allows oedema to form a pit when it is compressed by your thumb over the tibia (Fig. 12.2). Lymphoedema is non-pitting because the fluid is in lymphatic vessels and cannot move.

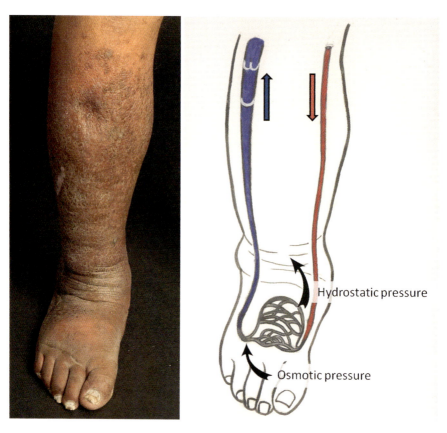

Fig. 12.1 The formation of oedema. Fluid is forced from the capillary bed at the arterial end by hydrostatic pressure and returns at the venous end by osmotic pressure

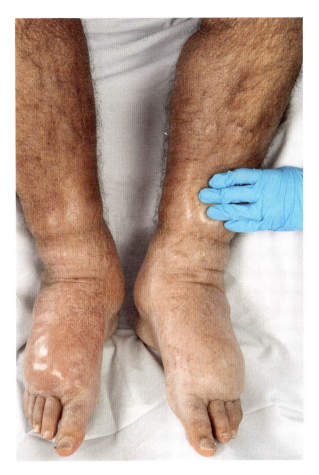

Fig. 12.2 This man has had nephrotic syndrome for a few weeks. The oedema is soft and pits easily with gentle pressure. An imprint of the fingers on the tibia is seen above the gloved hand

How Excess Salt and Water Can Be Removed

For oedema to be removed, salt excretion must exceed salt intake. As most drinks are hypotonic, imposing a limit on fluid intake – fluid restriction – is effectively water deprivation. This is either pointless, as the kidneys will counteract by concentrating the urine, or dangerous as it will eventually cause hypernatraemia.

Restricting salt intake may reduce oedema in chronic heart failure [2], although this is controversial [3], and helps to lower blood pressure and slow the decline in GFR in CKD [4].

The principal treatment of fluid overload is to increase salt excretion by the kidneys with diuretic drugs. The kidneys can only excrete salt and water that is in the plasma; interstitial fluid has to re-enter the plasma volume before it can be excreted. Ideally the rate of excretion from the plasma is in equilibrium with the rate of refilling of plasma from the interstitial fluid. Refilling from pleural effusions and ascites is slower than from the interstitial fluid.

In patients with nephrotic syndrome, hypoalbuminaemia lowers the low plasma osmotic pressure and slows the reabsorption of interstitial fluid. Plasma volume is more likely to fall when diuretics are given.

When salt and water are excreted faster than plasma volume is refilled, plasma volume is reduced and the reabsorption of glomerular filtrate by the tubules is increased. The flow of filtrate along the tubules is slowed, allowing more urea to diffuse out of the tubule into the plasma. This can be detected by an increase in the urea-to-creatinine ratio (see Sect. "Serum urea and creatinine – different measures of kidney function" in page 26).

Leg swelling typically increases during the day because venous pressure is increased by gravity. When the legs are raised to the level of the heart in bed at night, the oedema is reabsorbed, leading to nocturia.

Elderly people with heart failure may sleep in a chair rather than a bed because they get breathless if they lie flat. The venous return from their legs is continually exposed to gravity and fluid cannot leave the tissues. This can lead to chronic oedema and venous ulceration.

Similarly, in patients with high venous pressure due to right heart failure – cor pulmonale – oedema is harder to remove with diuretics and the urea-to-creatinine ratio is more likely to increase.

Assessing Fluid Balance in Acutely Ill Patients

Acute illness affects the excretion of salt and water and their distribution between body compartments:

• Cortisol production is increased leading to sodium and water retention
• Vasodilatation due to sepsis leads to low blood pressure
• Acute inflammation suppresses liver protein synthesis, so serum albumin concentration drops
• Acute inflammation weakens the capillary endothelial barrier, so fluid leaks into the interstitial space

When acute illness occurs in someone with chronic fluid overload, fluid balance is more difficult to assess. Blood pressure may be low due to reduced plasma volume despite there being peripheral oedema or ascites. Poor left ventricular function may contribute to the low blood pressure so giving intravenous fluid may risk causing pulmonary oedema.

Treatment with fluids and, if appropriate, antibiotics can be lifesaving and it is important to act promptly [5]. Tracking changes in vital signs and blood results helps in writing the fluid prescription (Patient 12.1).

Patient 12.1: Physiological Measurements in Acute Kidney Injury

Mr. Thomas, an 83-year-old retired machine operator, was admitted to a cardiac ward for investigation of recurrent blackouts. He was a lifelong smoker and hypertensive, treated with amlodipine.

On admission, urinalysis showed no blood or protein. U&E's and full blood count were normal.

During the night, about 24 h after admission, he complained of passing dark red urine in the toilet and became very anxious. Two hours later he became very unwell with a pulse rate of 170 beats per minute and collapsed to the floor, unresponsive and incontinent of faeces. Telemetry showed a prolonged period of supraventricular tachycardia.

His temperature was 40 °C, respiratory rate 44 breaths per minute, blood pressure 89/52 mmHg and pulse 150 beats per minute (Fig. 12.3). Arterial blood gases on 15 L per minute of oxygen showed: pO_2 20 kPa (11–13), pCO_2 3.98 kPa (4.7–6.0). There was a compensated metabolic acidosis: arterial pH 7.403 (normal 7.34–7.44), base excess = −5.7 mmol/L (−2 to +2), venous HCO_3^- = 9.6 mmol/L (22–26). Serum lactate was high: arterial sample = 7.4 mmol/L (0.5–1.6). White blood count was normal, 7.7×10^9/L.

He was resuscitated with 3 L of IV normal saline over the following 24 h. A urinary catheter was inserted and he was given intravenous broad-spectrum antibiotics pending the results of urine and blood cultures.

The next day his white count had jumped to 26.6×10^9/L. C-reactive protein increased to 176 mg/L and serum albumin dropped from 38 to 29 g/L (3.8–2.9 g/dL) – an acute phase reaction. A mid-stream urine specimen contained 115 WBC/microL (normal range 0–80) but culture yielded no growth. However, blood culture yielded *Escherichia coli,* fully sensitive to antibiotics.

His serum creatinine rose from a baseline of 82 micromol/L (0.9 mg/dL) to a peak of 268 micromol/L (3.0 mg/dL), a 227 % increase to 3.27 × baseline. Applying the KDIGO criteria, this is Stage 3 AKI (see Table 3.2).

During the first 24 h after the collapse his blood pressure was low, mean arterial pressure falling from 90 to 65 mmHg. During this period his kidney perfusion pressure fell below the level that could sustain glomerular filtration. He became oliguric for a period of 7 h.

Oliguria, defined as a urine volume of <400 ml per day or <0.5 ml/kg/h for more than 6 h, indicates an increased risk of mortality. Restoration of urine flow is a sign that GFR is recovering. As GFR increased, the slope of the serum creatinine graph switched from upwards to downwards (Fig. 12.4) eventually returning to his normal level.

Over 48 h Mr Thomas received a total of 7 L of intravenous normal saline. The period of low blood pressure was short, the infection was treated promptly and his circulation returned to normal [5]. Fluid given during resuscitation to restore the blood pressure was reabsorbed into the circulation and his urine volume increased – the diuretic phase.

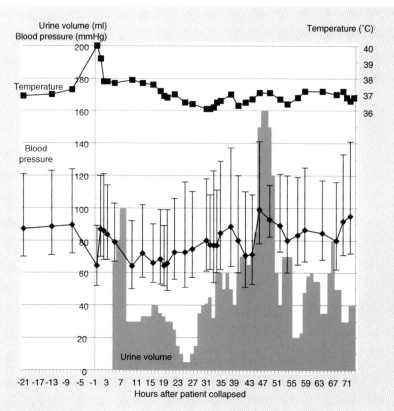

Fig. 12.3 Chart showing the vital signs for the 24 h before and 72 h after Mr Thomas' collapse due to sepsis

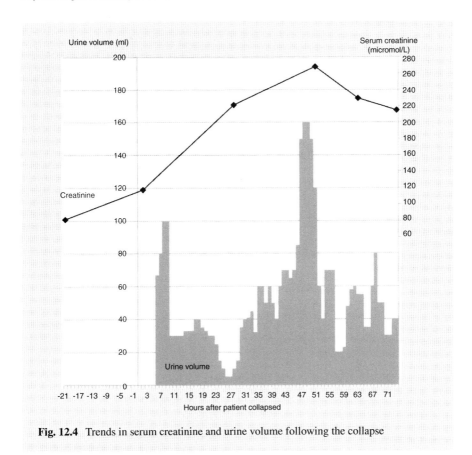

Fig. 12.4 Trends in serum creatinine and urine volume following the collapse

Physical Signs of Kidney Disease

Traditional physical signs of advanced kidney disease, such as uraemic frost and pigmentation, are rarely seen now that detection and treatment of kidney disease has improved.

Skin signs are usually related to systemic diseases that affect the kidneys. Vasculitis is the commonest and can have a range of appearances depending upon the size and location of the vessels affected (Figs. 12.5, 12.6, 12.7, and 12.8).

Fig. 12.5 Purpuric
vasculitic rash in a patient
with Henoch-Schönlein
Purpura

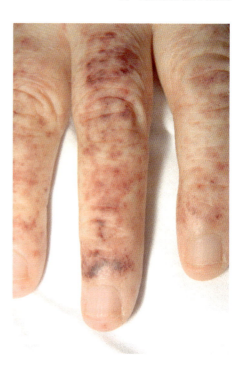

Fig. 12.6 Splinter
haemorrhages in a patient
with ANCA-associated
systemic necrotising
vasculitis

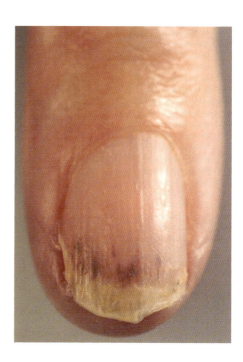

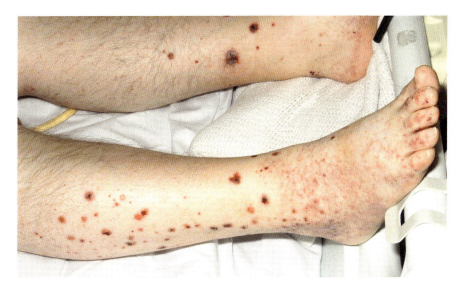

Fig. 12.7 Vasculitic and purpuric rash affecting the legs of a patient with Henoch-Schönlein purpura. Skin biopsy showed a leucocytoclastic vasculitis

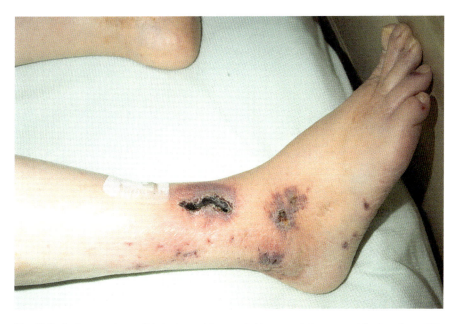

Fig. 12.8 Oedema and vasculitic lesions with central skin necrosis in a man with ulcerative colitis and antiphospholipid syndrome. He also suffered a bowel infarction requiring total colectomy. The dressing covers the wound from a skin biopsy that showed a vasculitic process with fibrin thrombi affecting all the vessels

Examine the Abdomen

If you are able to feel a kidney by bimanual palpation, it is enlarged. This may be due to a tumour, gross hydronephrosis or polycystic kidney disease.

In patients with hypertension, it is traditional to listen for an abdominal bruit. Systolic bruits are frequently heard over the aorta or femoral arteries. In someone with atherosclerotic vascular disease, a bruit heard in both systole and diastole suggests renovascular disease (see Sect. "Atherosclerosis" in page 67) [6].

It is always worth examining for an enlarged bladder. Chronic retention of urine can develop without the patient recognising anything is wrong (see Patient 3.4: Interpreting a more complex eGFR graph). The bladder may not be tense but is stony dull to percussion. It is easy to measure the volume using an ultrasound bladder scanner (Fig. 12.9).

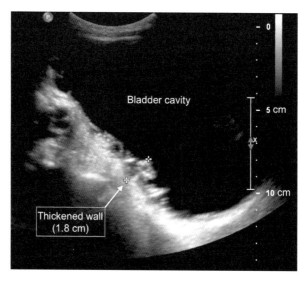

Fig. 12.9 Ultrasound scan of a patient with chronic bladder outflow obstruction. The bladder is distended and the wall is thickened with an irregular trabeculated surface. In a man, these appearances are usually caused by prostatic enlargement. These images are from a woman with a urethral stricture

References

1. Fortes MB, Owen JA, Raymond-Barker P, Bishop C, Elghenzai S, Oliver SJ, Walsh NP. Is this elderly patient dehydrated? diagnostic accuracy of hydration assessment using physical signs, urine, and saliva markers. J Am Med Direct Assoc. 2015;16(3):221–8. http://www.ncbi.nlm.nih.gov/pubmed/25444573.

2. Philipson H, Ekman I, Forslund HB, Swedberg K, Schaufelberger M. Salt and fluid restriction is effective in patients with chronic heart failure. Eur J Heart Fail. 2013;15(11)):1304–10. doi:10.1093/eurjhf/hft097. Epub 2013 Jun 19. http://onlinelibrary.wiley.com/doi/10.1093/eur-jhf/hft097/full.

3. Konerman MC, Hummel SL. Sodium restriction in heart failure: benefit or harm? Curr Treat Options Cardiovasc Med. 2014;16(2):286. doi:10.1007/s11936-013-0286-x. http://www.ncbi.nlm.nih.gov/pmc/articles/PMC3947770/.

4. Vegter S, Perna A, Postma MJ, Navis G, Remuzzi G, Ruggenenti P. Sodium intake, ACE inhibition, and progression to ESRD. J Am Soc Nephrol. 2012;23(1):165–73. doi:10.1681/ASN.2011040430. Epub 2011 Dec 1. http://jasn.asnjournals.org/content/23/1/165.long.

5. Mouncey PR, Osborn TM, Power GS, Harrison DA, Sadique MZ, Grieve RD, Jahan R, Harvey SE, Bell D, Bion JF, Coats TJ, Singer M, Young JD, Rowan KM, ProMISe Trial Investigators. Trial of early, goal-directed resuscitation for septic shock. New Eng J Med. 2015. doi:10.1056/NEJMoa1500896. http://www.nejm.org/doi/pdf/10.1056/NEJMoa1500896.

6. Krijnen P, van Jaarsveld BC, Steyerberg EW, Veld AJ M i 't, Schalekamp MA, Habbema JD. A clinical prediction rule for renal artery stenosis. Ann Intern Med. 1998;129(9):705–11. http://annals.org/article.aspx?articleid=711773.

Chapter 13
Full Blood Count, Urea and Electrolytes, Bicarbonate, Bone Profile

Laboratory Results and Kidney Diseases

Abstract In this chapter we explain:

- Anaemia due to kidney disease
- Kidney disease linked to causes of anaemia
- The importance of acidosis in chronic kidney disease
- Effects of kidney failure on bone and mineral metabolism
- Hyperparathyroidism and the effects of parathyroidectomy
- How hypercalcaemia is linked to kidney disease

As kidney function declines, three main laboratory test abnormalities develop (Fig. 13.1).

- Low Hb – anaemia
- Low serum bicarbonate – acidosis
- Low calcium and raised phosphate and PTH – mineral bone disease

Anaemia

Erythropoietin and the Regulation of Haemoglobin

Anaemia in kidney disease is due to insufficient production of erythropoietin combined with a shortening of the life span of red blood cells.

Erythropoietin increases the production of red cells by binding to specific receptors on erythroid progenitor cells in the bone marrow, triggering a cascade of intracellular protein phosphorylations. As a consequence of this activation, the cells proceed to form mature red cells rather than undergo apoptosis.

In the fetus and newborn babies, erythropoietin is produced predominantly by the liver. In infancy production shifts to the kidneys as their blood flow and function increases. In adults, 90 % of erythropoietin comes from the kidneys.

© Springer International Publishing Switzerland 2016
H. Rayner et al., *Understanding Kidney Diseases*,
DOI 10.1007/978-3-319-23458-8_13

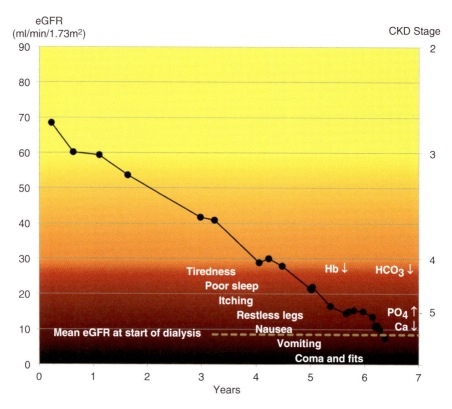

Fig. 13.1 Laboratory test abnormalities and symptoms that occur at different stages of chronic kidney disease

Erythropoietin production is controlled by changes in the pressure of oxygen (pO_2) dissolved in tissue fluid. The oxygen sensing takes place inside interstitial fibroblast cells, located between the tubules in the deep layers of the renal cortex close to the peritubular capillaries [1].

The control of erythropoietin production is mediated by hypoxia-inducible factors (HIFs), which promote transcription of the erythropoietin gene. When pO_2 is normal, HIF is rapidly hydroxylated by oxygen-dependent HIF prolyl-4-hydroxylase domain (PHD) enzymes and so does not accumulate in the interstitial cell. Under hypoxic conditions the PHD enzymes are not activated; HIF levels increase in the cell and turn on the erythropoietin gene. Erythropoietin levels in blood may increase 1000-fold in anaemia not related to CKD.

As GFR drops, the haemoglobin concentration falls (Patient 13.1). The reduction in erythropoietin production in kidney disease is due to reduced responsiveness of the interstitial cells to hypoxia from reduced HIF activity, combined with a reduced capacity to produce erythropoietin. If HIF levels are increased by pharmacological inhibition of the PHD enzymes, erythropoietin production increases [2].

Patient 13.1: The Development of Anaemia in Chronic Kidney Disease
Mr. Roberts was under regular follow up for CKD and hypertension. Over the course of a year his eGFR dropped further, by half. An ultrasound scan showed a shrunken right kidney.

As the right kidney atrophied, glomerular filtration and erythropoetin production declined, leading to a decline in eGFR and haemoglobin concentration (Fig. 13.2).

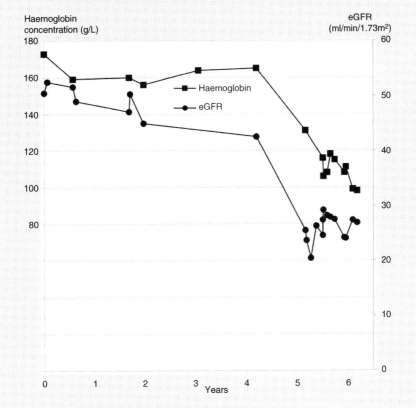

Fig. 13.2 Parallel reductions in eGFR and haemoglobin concentration due to atrophy of one kidney in a patient with pre-existing chronic kidney disease

Why in the Kidneys?

Why are the kidneys central to the regulation of red cell production by the bone marrow? The answer to this question becomes clear from thinking about the role of haemoglobin in survival and evolution.

The optimal haemoglobin (Hb) concentration is the one that delivers oxygen most efficiently to the tissues. Too high a concentration increases the risk of hyperviscosity and clotting and too low risks high output cardiac failure. The regulatory mechanism maintains a basal rate of red cell production to replace red cells that are cleared from the circulation at the end of their life. When the Hb concentration falls below the optimum level, the regulatory mechanism stimulates red cell production.

A low Hb concentration provides an inadequate supply of O_2 to the tissues. This may be compensated by an increase in blood flow, for example in exercising muscles by up to 20-fold. Tissues that are unable to compensate for anaemia by increasing their blood flow are vulnerable to hypoxic damage.

Kidney blood flow has to be closely regulated. If the blood flow rate increased in response to anaemia, GFR would also increase. This would increase the amount of O_2 and energy required by the tubules to reabsorb the increased amount of filtered sodium. The increased O_2 consumption would negate the extra O_2 provided by the increased blood flow.

Because hypoxia cannot be compensated by increased blood flow, the kidneys are at risk of hypoxic damage due to anaemia. Locating the haemoglobin regulatory mechanism in the region of the kidney most at risk – the deep cortex – provides the greatest survival advantage.

The anaemia of CKD provides some survival advantage against cardiovascular disease. Blood clotting is impaired due to anaemia and impaired platelet function. The risk of stroke increases if the anaemia is corrected with recombinant erythropoietin [3].

Anaemia has also indirectly increased survival from renal failure through dialysis. The success of haemodialysis is possible because of the arterio-venous fistula that allows repeated safe access to the circulation (see Sect. "Vascular access" in page 255). If one attempts to create a fistula in someone with normal kidney function, the vein clots almost immediately. Similarly, if a dialysis patient regains normal kidney function with a transplant, the fistula usually clots. The anaemia and bleeding tendency of renal failure have permitted the evolution of haemodialysis by allowing arterio-venous fistulas to function.

The red cells are normal in CKD – the anaemia is normochromic normocytic – and the other cells lines are normal. If someone with CKD has abnormal red cells or changes in white cells or platelets, an alternative cause for the anaemia should be sought. Common causes include iron deficiency from gastrointestinal blood loss or coeliac disease and folate or vitamin B12 deficiency causing macrocytic anaemia.

Kidney Disease Linked to Causes of Anaemia

The cause of the anaemia may sometimes also be the cause of the kidney disease. Sickle cell anaemia is common; paroxysmal nocturnal haemoglobinuria (PNH) and haemolytic uraemic syndrome (HUS) are rare. In all three, anaemia is caused by intravascular haemolysis. If haemolysis is suspected, check for a raised serum lactate dehydrogenase (LDH), which is released from the red cells.

Sickle cell anaemia can cause infarction of the renal medulla and papillae through sickling of red cells in this hypoxic region. Necrotic papillae slough off into the pelvis and can cause haematuria, ureteric colic and obstruction.

Chronic medullary ischaemia causes haematuria and impairs the kidney's ability to concentrate urine and excrete acid and potassium. Patients may have a wide range of clinical presentations including haematuria, proteinuria, nephrotic syndrome, acute and chronic kidney disease. The pathological mechanisms underlying many of these complications remain unclear [4].

Paroxysmal nocturnal haemoglobinuria (PNH) is caused by an acquired defect of protective proteins on the red cell membrane – a deficiency of glycophosphatidylinositol. It may occur in isolation or as part of a bone marrow disorder such as aplastic anemia. Only a quarter of patients have red urine (haemoglobinuria) in the morning. It may present with acute or chronic kidney disease due to haemoglobin occluding or damaging tubules and stimulating interstitial fibrosis [5]. It may be treated with eculizumab, a monoclonal antibody that inhibits the complement activation that attacks the red cell membrane (see Fig. 14.4).

Haemolytic uraemic syndrome (**HUS**) is divided into two forms: typical diarrhoea-positive (D+ HUS) and atypical (aHUS).

D+ HUS is the consequence of an infection, usually due to *Escherichia coli* subtype O157. The infection is typically contracted from undercooked beef, contaminated dairy products or contact with the organism in the environment such as petting farms.

The *E. coli* produces a shiga-like toxin, also known as verocytotoxin, which damages endothelial cells, activates neutrophils and triggers the coagulation pathway. This consumes platelets and causes a microangiopathic haemolytic anaemia (MAHA) (Fig. 13.3).

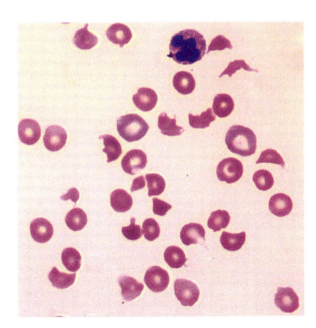

Fig. 13.3 Blood film showing microangiopathic haemolytic anaemia. There are large numbers of fragmented and abnormally shaped red cells called schistocytes indicating damage to red cell membranes, and low numbers of platelets

Fig. 13.4 Section of a glomerulus from a patient with HUS showing glomerular capillaries containing microthrombi and red cells (*arrow*). Haematoxylin and eosin ×60

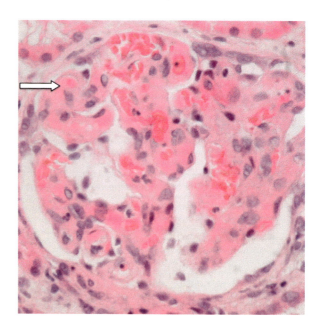

Microthromi occlude the glomerular capillaries, causing acute kidney injury (Fig. 13.4).

Once the acute illness is passed, the glomerular microthrombi resolve and the capillaries reopen. Hence treatment of the condition is supportive, about 50 % of patients requiring dialysis, usually for up to 2 weeks (Patient 13.2).

Patient 13.2: Typical Diarrhoea-Positive (D+ HUS)

Ten-year-old Rosie was admitted to hospital with a 3-day history of diarrhea, with blood for the last 24 h. She had drunk unpasteurised milk 4 days before the diarrhoea. Serum electrolytes and creatinine were normal for her age (creatinine 50 micromol/L = 0.6 mg/dL). Haemoglobin was increased due to acute dehydration (174 g/L = 17.4 g/dL). Neutrophils were raised (17.7 × 10^9/L) but platelets and clotting were normal. She was given oral rehydration mixture.

Two days later serum sodium had fallen to 130 mmol/L, creatinine increased to 345 micromol/L (3.9 mg/dL). Haemoglobin had fallen to 117 g/L (11.7 g/dL) and platelets to 76 × 10^9/L. Stool culture grew *Escherichia coli* O157.

Over the next 5 days her creatinine rose to 975 micromol/L (11.0 mg/dL) and she commenced peritoneal dialysis, which continued for 13 days. Her haemoglobin fell further to 74 g/L (7.4 g/dL) and the film showed fragmented red cells typical of microangiopathic haemolytic anaemia. She was given a blood transfusion.

Two months later her creatinine had returned to her normal level and she has since remained well.

aHUS is atypical in that there is usually no or only mild diarrhoea and no *E. coli* infection. Hypertension is common and can be severe. Up to 70 % progress to end-stage kidney failure and there is a high risk of recurrence after a kidney transplant.

The condition can present at any age, 60 % in childhood. It may be familial and up to 80 % of cases have genetic abnormalities of complement regulation (Patient 13.3).

When the condition involves other organs, notably the nervous system with seizures and coma, it is termed thrombotic thrombocytopenic purpura-hemolytic uremic syndrome (TTP-HUS). Patients with TTP classically have severe deficiency of ADAMTS13, the von Willebrand factor-cleaving protease. ADAMTS13 normally breaks down multimers of von Willebrand factor, reducing their clotting activity [6].

Treatment traditionally involved plasmapheresis and FFP infusions but had a rate of dialysis or death of 40 %. The monoclonal antibody eculizumab is now used because the condition, like PNH, is mediated by the complement cascade (see Sect. "Complement C3 and C4" in page 202).

Patient 13.3: Atypical HUS (aHUS)

Peter, aged 5, was admitted with a 3-day history of vomiting, jaundice and abdominal cramps without diarrhoea. He was pale, icteric and had petechiae on his limbs and trunk. Blood count confirmed low haemoglobin with fragmented red blood cells on the film. Serum lactate dehydrogenase and creatinine were raised (Fig. 13.5).

His older brother had had an episode of low platelets and transient anaemia at the age of 5 years, diagnosed as thrombotic thrombocytopenic purpura, and had made a full recovery.

A diagnosis of atypical HUS was made and Peter was treated with daily plasma exchange. His kidney function and blood count recovered quickly. He was maintained on regular plasmapheresis and then eculizumab infusions every 2 weeks.

Genetic studies identified a mutation of the CD46 membrane cofactor protein gene in both Peter and his brother. This cofactor degrades complement components C3b and C4b, interrupting the complement cascade. Loss of its function leads to unregulated formation of the complement membrane attack complex that causes endothelial cell damage (see Fig. 14.4).

Eculizumab infusions were discontinued after 6 months but he was admitted 9 months later with a recurrence of HUS (Fig. 13.5). This responded rapidly to eculizumab alone and he remains on 3 weekly infusions.

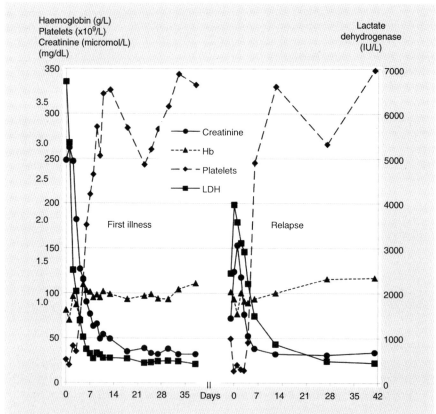

Fig. 13.5 Patterns of creatinine, blood count and lactate dehydrogenase (LDH) during two episodes of aHUS

Acid, Base, Bicarbonate and Total CO₂

A simple indicator of acid-base balance in kidney disease is the concentration of bicarbonate in a venous serum sample. The laboratory may measure the serum total CO_2 content instead of bicarbonate. Total CO_2 includes bicarbonate ions, dissolved CO_2 and carbonic acid. Bicarbonate comprises about 95 % of the total CO_2 content.

Acid is mainly excreted in the urine as ammonium ions (NH_4^+). The smell of stale urine comes from the breakdown of ammonium chloride and urea to ammonia. In Roman times, stale urine was collected and used for cleaning and for whitening teeth.

As the number of working nephrons declines, ammonium excretion per remaining nephron increases. This is mediated through increased angiotensin production by the kidney. When GFR falls below about 45 ml/min/1/73 m^2, total ammonium excretion starts to fall. Initially, excess H$^+$ ions are buffered by bicarbonate in the extracellular fluid and by tissue buffers and bone. But as GFR falls further, these buffers become saturated, metabolic acidosis develops and serum bicarbonate falls.

The acidosis is not only a consequence of the loss of GFR; it also contributes to its progression [7]. The risk of GFR declining is associated with the level of serum bicarbonate, the lower the level the greater the risk. This association is found over a range of serum bicarbonate that includes normal values, that is above 22 mmol/l.

Randomised controlled trials of patients with CKD stages 3 or below and serum bicarbonate <24 mmol/L have shown that treatment with oral sodium bicarbonate or a diet high in alkali-producing fruits and vegetables significantly reduces the rate of decline in GFR and the chances of starting dialysis over the following 2–3 years.

The mechanism of this important effect is mediated by a reduction in production of angiotensin II in the kidney, measured by the level of angiotensinogen in the urine [8].

Bicarbonate treatment also increases protein intake and reduces the impact of acidosis on protein breakdown. Treated patients have better nutritional status, such as mid-arm circumference and serum albumin [9]. Sodium bicarbonate does not cause signs of sodium overload such as oedema or high blood pressure; in this respect, sodium bicarbonate behaves differently to sodium chloride.

Increasing dietary acid intake in the form of two or more cola drinks a day, which contain phosphoric acid, is associated with a doubling of the risk of chronic kidney disease [10].

Vitamin D, Minerals, Bones and Blood Vessels

Serum phosphate is derived predominantly from the catabolism of phosphorylated proteins. As GFR declines, the excretion of phosphate decreases. Eventually excretion fails to balance production and serum phosphate increases. This is exemplified in Patient 13.4.

Patient 13.4: Development of Abnormal Mineral Metabolism in Chronic Kidney Disease
Mr. Jordan, a fit 65-year-old white man, had IgA nephropathy. His eGFR declined by more than 15 ml/min/1.73 m^2/year and he showed typical changes in serum calcium, phosphate and parathyroid hormone (PTH) (Fig. 13.6). He did not take any calcium or vitamin D supplements during this time.

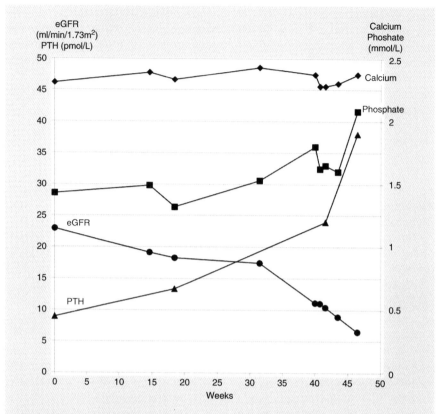

Fig. 13.6 Trends in serum calcium, phosphate and parathyroid hormone (PTH) as GFR declines. To convert units: calcium 2.5 mmol/L = 10.0 mg/dL; phosphate 2 mmol/L = phosphorus 6.2 mg/dL; PTH 50 pmol/L = 470 pg/ml

Figure 13.6 shows how parathyroid hormone (PTH) increases as the eGFR decreases. The main function of PTH is to regulate the serum calcium concentration. A fall in serum calcium is detected by the calcium-sensing receptors on the chief cells of the parathyroid glands, triggering an increase in PTH production and secretion. PTH stimulates calcium absorption from the gut and release from bone. The basic elements of the feedback control of serum calcium and phosphate are shown in Fig. 13.7.

But Mr Jordan's calcium showed no sign of decreasing, so why was the PTH high?

PTH is normally suppressed both by calcium and by activated vitamin D (Fig. 13.7) and the main cause of the increase in PTH in CKD is a decrease in vitamin D activity.

Vitamin D_3 (cholecalciferol) is synthesized in the deeper layers of the skin and absorbed from the gut. In the liver it is converted to the storage form of vitamin D_3, 25(OH)-vitamin D_3. It is activated by 1-hydroxylation to 1,25(OH)$_2$-vitamin D_3

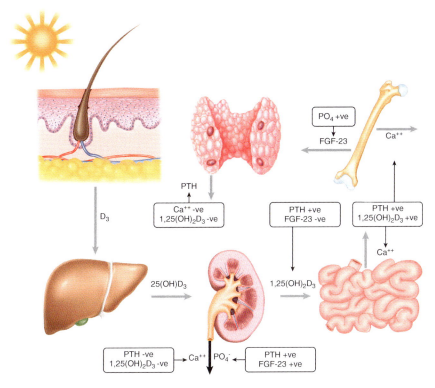

Fig. 13.7 The main components of feedback control of serum calcium and phosphate. The white arrows indicate the source of substances, released into the circulation. The black arrow indicates excretion into the urine. Feedback is shown in boxes, either negative (suppression) or positive (stimulation). D_3 = vitamin D_3. $1,25(OH)_2D_3$ = calcitriol

(calcitriol). This occurs in many tissues but the main source of systemically active calcitriol is the kidneys.

CKD leads to reduced calcitriol production through a number of mechanisms [11]. Firstly, patients often lack sufficient 25(OH)-vitamin D_3 from diet and sun exposure, especially in dark skinned races. Secondly, reduced GFR and damage to tubular cells limit the capacity for 25(OH)-vitamin D_3 to be hydroxylated in the renal cortex.

Thirdly, high serum phosphate levels stimulate the release of factors that increase urinary phosphate excretion called phosphatonins. These include fibroblast growth factor 23 (FGF-23), which is produced by bone osteoblasts, filtered by glomeruli and broken down in proximal tubules. The interaction between FGF-23, vitamin D_3 and PTH is complicated [12].

In CKD, FGF-23 increases and suppresses 1-alpha-hydroxylase activity, leading to deficiency of calcitriol.

Because PTH production is normally suppressed by vitamin D_3, low levels of calcitriol allow PTH production to increase – secondary hyperparathyroidism. The increased PTH in turn stimulates 1-alpha-hydroxylase activity in the proximal tubules, boosting calcitriol production, and increases osteoclast activity in bone to release calcium. Both these actions mitigate against a drop in serum calcium in CKD, as shown in Patient 13.2.

Calcitriol increases absorption of calcium from the intestines and from the renal tubules. It is also required for the coupling of osteoblast and osteoclast function in bone remodelling. Persistent calcitriol deficiency in CKD eventually leads to hypocalcaemia.

Why Is Vitamin D Activated in the Kidneys?

It may seem odd that the kidneys are the main site of activation of vitamin D in the body. As with the regulation of haemoglobin being located in the kidney (see Sect. "Why in the kidneys?" in page 175), the explanation comes from the pressures of evolution.

Free vitamin D is a steroid and so can diffuse freely across cell membranes. To avoid it being lost from the circulation and to enable its uptake into cells to be actively controlled, it is almost all bound to a plasma protein, Vitamin D-Binding Protein (DBP). DBP is small enough (58 kDa, compared to albumin 66.5 kDa) to be filtered by the glomerulus in significant amounts.

If filtered vitamins were lost into the urine, severe vitamin D deficiency, hypocalcaemia and bone disease would develop. This can be produced experimentally in genetically modified mice and occurs naturally in some types of Fanconi syndrome (see Table 7.1) [13].

To avoid this loss, filtered 25(OH)-vitamin D_3 bound to DBP is taken up by proximal tubular cells. Once inside the mitochondria of these cells, the 25(OH)-vitamin D_3 is hydroxylated to the active form, calcitriol, which is then bound to DBP and released into the circulation. By combining the conservation and activation of vitamin D into one uptake process in the kidneys, survival is ensured using the minimum amount of metabolic energy.

Hyperparathyroidism

Progressive enlargement of the parathyroid glands tends to occur in patients with long-standing CKD despite treatment with vitamin D supplements and dietary phosphate binders. Persistently high PTH levels increase bone turnover. The volume of unmineralised bone is increased, with more osteoclasts and osteoblasts – renal osteodystrophy. The bone structure is weakened and may fracture (Patient 13.5).

High PTH levels combined with persistent hyperphosphataemia in CKD stages 4 and 5 lead to the deposition of calcium and phosphate in blood vessels and other tissues. This contributes to an increased risk of cardiovascular disease.

Patient 13.5: Severe Hyperparathyroidism

Mrs. Bibi had advanced chronic kidney disease due to kidney stones for over 25 years. For the last 10 years she had been treated with haemodialysis. The serum alkaline phosphatase had progressively risen to over 1000 IU/L (normal range 30–130) and parathyroid hormone to 452 pmol/L (normal 1.6–6.9; =4262 pg/ml). She had declined parathyroid surgery.

She was admitted with severe pain in the legs. A plain X-ray was taken (Fig. 13.8).

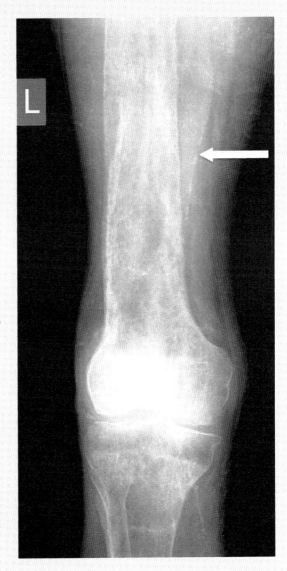

Fig. 13.8 Plain X-ray showing severe renal osteodystrophy affecting the femur, tibia and fibula. The bone texture is very abnormal with loss of mineral density, destruction of the normal trabeculae and subperiosteal erosions. There is calcification in the femoral artery (*arrow*)

Soon afterwards, she suffered a pathological fracture of the femur.

A year later, she was admitted with difficulty speaking and swallowing. A CT scan of the skull showed thickening and abnormal texture of the bones, particularly affecting the jaw and facial bones. At the base of the skull at the right antero-lateral aspect of the foreman magnum there was a 2.1 × 3.7 cm brown tumour. This is composed of fibrous tissue and unmineralised woven bone, and is coloured brown by haemosiderin deposition. It had caused pressure on the spinal cord and lower cranial nerves (Fig. 13.9).

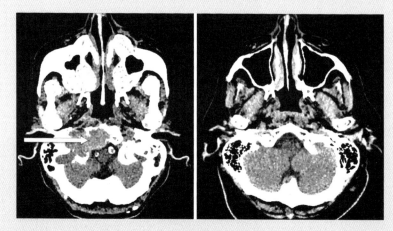

Fig. 13.9 CT scan of the base of the skull showing (*left*) massive hypertrophy of the facial bones and a tumour at the foramen magnum compressing the brain stem (*arrow*). There is also calcification in the vertebral and scalp arteries. A normal scan is shown for comparison (*right*)

Parathyroidectomy

Prolonged stimulation of the parathyroid glands can lead to one or more parathyroid hormone-producing cells becoming unresponsive to the suppressive effect of serum calcium. One cell in each gland may multiply to form an adenoma made up of clones of cells. These adenomata are autonomous, i.e., they secrete large amounts of PTH despite the serum calcium being normal. Eventually the serum calcium is elevated – tertiary hyperparathyroidism.

A drug that mimics the effect of calcium on the calcium sensing receptors on the parathyroid cells, the calcimimetic cinacalcet, can be used to lower PTH and serum calcium. However, it does not provide a clear clinical benefit in bone health or cardiovascular outcomes in patients on dialysis [14]. Conversely, parathyroidectomy – the surgical removal of all the enlarged glands – is associated with a 34–43 % reduction in subsequent mortality in patients with severe hyperparathyroidism [15, 16].

After parathyroidectomy, there is a sudden drop in PTH and osteoclast activity. Bone mineral resorption and release of calcium stops but bone formation continues. Large quantities of calcium re-enter the skeleton from the blood – the 'hungry bone' syndrome. Rapid and severe hypocalcaemia can occur, the severity being proportional to the pre-operative alkaline phosphatase, which reflects the 'appetite' of the bones.

Over the following weeks the alkaline phosphatase rises as osteoblast activity increases and then falls as the bones are satiated with calcium. This trend can be used to guide the dosage of calcium and vitamin D supplements to keep the serum calcium within the normal range (Patient 13.6).

Patient 13.6: The Effects of Parathyroidectomy on Calcium Metabolism
Sally had been on dialysis for 10 years. Despite treatment with the calcimi-metic drug cinacalcet, her hyperparathyroidism had progressed to a tertiary stage, i.e., hypercalcaemia with a high PTH. She had aching pains in her hips, knees and feet.

In November 2011, what appeared to be four enlarged parathyroid glands were surgically removed. However, histological examination showed one to be lymphoid tissue. Her serum calcium and PTH remained elevated.

A nuclear medicine parathyroid subtraction scan was performed. In this procedure, a radioisotope, technetium 99 m pertechnetate, is injected and taken up by the thyroid gland. This is followed by an injection of technetium 99 m sestamibi that is taken up by both thyroid and parathyroid glands (Fig. 13.10).

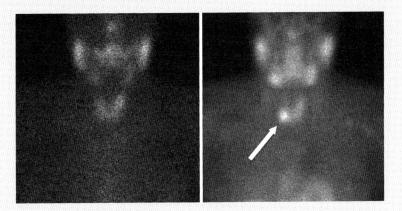

Fig. 13.10 Technetium 99 m (99mTc) pertechnetate scan (*left*) showing the thyroid gland and laryngeal bones. Technetium 99 m sestamibi (MIBI) scan (*right*) shows a hot spot at the lower pole of the right lobe of thyroid (*arrow*)

Subtracting one scan from the other reveals the parathyroid gland (Fig. 13.11).

In August 2012, a further operation was performed to remove the fourth gland. The effect on her blood results is shown in Fig. 13.12.

Removal of the remaining overactive gland led to an abrupt drop in serum PTH, calcium and phosphate. The alkaline phosphatase initially rose and then declined exponentially as bone turnover returned to a normal rate.

In September, 6 weeks after the operation, when alkaline phosphatase approached the normal range (30–130 IU/L), the dose of elemental calcium and then of $1\alpha(OH)$-vitamin D_3 (alfacalcidol) was reduced to avoid hypercalcaemia. Subsequent adjustments in the dose of alfacalcidol were too large, causing swings in serum calcium outside the normal range.

A stable equilibrium was reached 6 months after the operation. Sally's bone pains resolved and she felt generally much better.

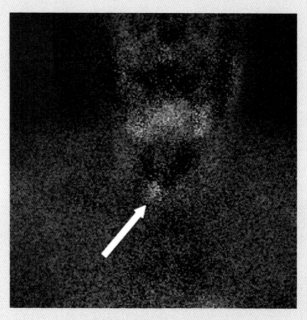

Fig. 13.11 99mTc + MIBI subtraction scan showing a hot spot (*arrow*) consistent with a right lower pole parathyroid adenoma

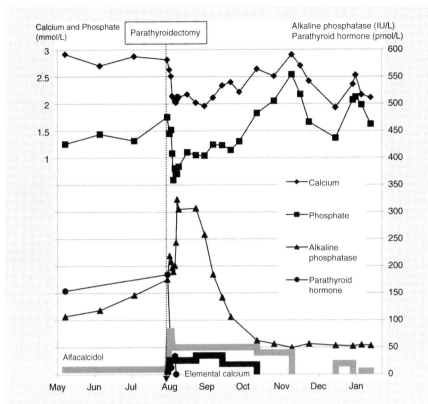

Fig. 13.12 Changes in bone biochemistry after parathyroidectomy. To convert units: calcium 2.5 mmol/L = 10.0 mg/dL; phosphate 2 mmol/L = phosphorus 6.2 mg/dL; PTH 300 pmol/L = 2800 pg/ml

Hypercalcaemia

It takes years for hypercalcaemia to develop as a result of kidney failure, as in Sally's case (Patient 13.6). If serum calcium is raised when kidney disease is first discovered, the hypercalcaemia is likely to be causing the reduced GFR or be due to the disease that is causing the kidney damage.

High serum calcium, particularly over 3 mmol/L (12 mg/dL), reduces GFR by causing vasoconstriction within the kidney [17]. It can also reduce the ability of the tubules to concentrate urine and so cause dehydration.

The first thing to check is the medication list. Hypercalcaemia may be caused by excessive calcium and vitamin D treatment. Thiazide diuretics reduce calcium excretion by the distal tubule and can cause mild hypercalaemia.

Table 13.1 Causes of hypercalcaemia that also affect kidney function

	Cause of hypercalcaemia	Cause of reduced GFR other than hypercalcaemia
Malignancy (Patient 13.7)	Calcium released from bone by osteolytic deposits and/or PTH-related peptide	Urinary tract obstruction
Primary hyperparathyroidism	PTH-producing adenoma not suppressed by serum calcium	Kidney stones nephrocalcinosis
Multiple myeloma (see Sect. "Immunoglobulins, protein electrophoresis, free light chains in serum and urine" in page 198)	Calcium released from bone by osteolytic deposits	Casts of paraprotein blocking tubules
Sarcoidosis (Patient 13.8)	$1,25(OH)_2$-vitamin D_3 produced by granulomas	Granulomas infiltrating the kidney interstitium

Diseases which cause hypercalcaemia can also reduce GFR in other ways. These are listed in Table 13.1.

Patient 13.7: Hypercalcaemia Due to Malignancy Causing Acute Kidney Injury

Mrs. Reynolds, aged 60 years, was admitted to hospital with pain in the left hip. She had had a squamous cell carcinoma of the mouth treated with chemo-radiotherapy a year previously. Three months before admission, serum urea and electrolytes were normal.

Laboratory results on admission showed acute kidney injury and severe hypercalcaemia (Table 13.2)

A urinary tract ultrasound scan was normal.

Plain X-ray of the left femur and pelvis showed a lytic lesion in the inferior pubic ramus (Fig. 13.13), confirmed by CT scan (Fig. 13.14). Biopsy showed it to be a secondary deposit.

Table 13.2 Laboratory results on admission to hospital

		Normal range	Non-SI units
Sodium	139 mmol/L	133–146	139 mEq/L
Potassium	3.5 mmol/L	3.5–5.3	3.5 mEq/L
Urea	31.2 mmol/L	2.5–7.8	BUN 87 mg/dL
Creatinine	475 micromol/L	64–111	5.4 mg/dL
eGFR	8 ml/min/1.73 m^2		
Albumin	29 g/L	35–50	2.9 g/dL
Calcium (corrected for serum albumin)	4.12 mmol/L	2.20–2.60	16.5 mg/dL
Phosphate	2.00 mmol/L	0.80–1.50	Phosphorus 6.2 mg/dL
Alkaline phosphatase	71 IU/L	30–130	

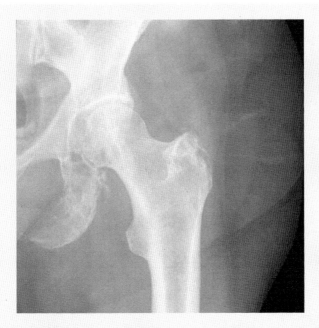

Fig. 13.13 Plain X-ray of the left femur and pelvis showing a lytic lesion in the inferior pubic ramus

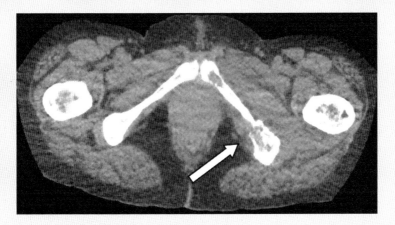

Fig. 13.14 CT scan showing a soft-tissue swelling beside the lesion, consistent with a metastatic deposit (*arrow*)

Patient 13.8: Hypercalcaemia Due to Sarcoidosis Causing Acute Kidney Injury

Ian, a 38-year-old businessman, first presented to his GP having felt generally tried and unwell for a few weeks. He was noted to have red eyes and swollen lymph nodes. It was thought he most likely had a viral infection but his renal function was reduced, eGFR = 30 ml/min/1.73 m^2. This improved to 60 ml/min/1.73 m^2 over the subsequent 10 weeks and he felt much better. He was referred to the haematology clinic for assessment of the lymphadenopathy.

The serum calcium level was elevated, 2.71 mmol/l (10.8 mg/dL). An ultrasound scan showed normal-sized kidneys but very prominent renal pyramids (Fig. 13.15).

A CT scan of the thorax and abdomen revealed widespread bulky lymphadenopathy in the neck, chest and upper abdomen, particularly the anterior mediastinum (Fig. 13.16).

Sarcoidosis was considered likely but lymphoma needed to be excluded, so a lymph node biopsy was performed. Histology showed tightly packed small granulomas composed of epithelioid histiocytes with no necrosis. The residual lymphoid tissue consisted of lymphocytes and mature plasma cells with no atypical cells. These features are consistent with sarcoidosis (Fig. 13.17).

The serum angiotensin-converting enzyme (ACE) was markedly raised at 226 IU/l (normal range 20–70). ACE is produced by granulomas and, when combined with other features, supports a diagnosis of sarcoidosis.

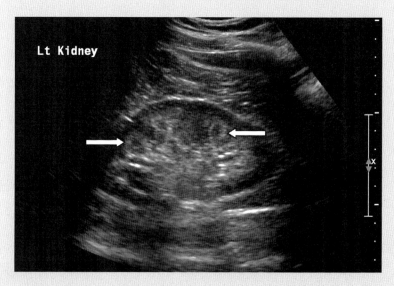

Fig. 13.15 Ultrasound scan of the left kidney showing prominent renal pyramids (*arrows*), consistent with infiltration or possible papillary necrosis

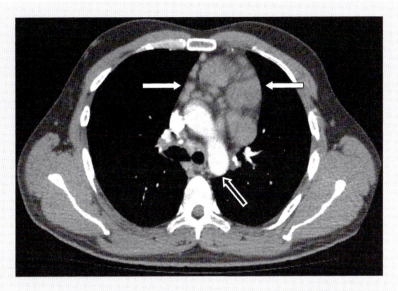

Fig. 13.16 Contrast CT scan section at the level of the aortic arch (enhanced with contrast *black arrow*), showing massively enlarged lymph nodes in the anterior mediastinum (*white arrows*)

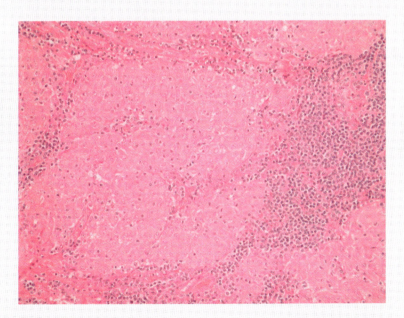

Fig. 13.17 Light micrograph of the excised lymph node showing compact coalescing granulomas with intervening lymphoid tissue, H&E ×200

Ian was feeling completely well. However, serial eGFR measurements showed that his kidney function was worsening again. He was therefore started on 10 mg of prednisolone per day. Over the subsequent months, his serum ACE steadily declined to normal, the size of the lymph nodes in his chest reduced slightly on a repeat CT scan, and serum calcium and renal function returned to normal (Fig. 13.18).

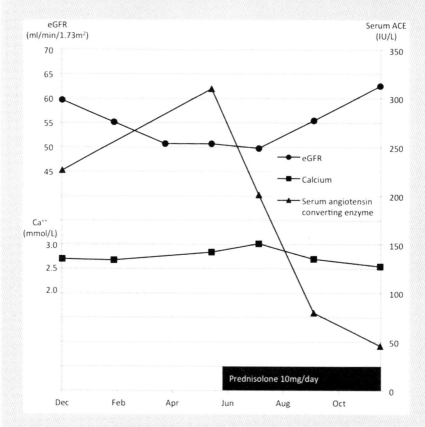

Fig. 13.18 Changes in eGFR, serum calcium and serum ACE with steroid therapy in sarcoidosis. To convert units: calcium 2.5 mmol/L = 10.0 mg/dL

References

1. Zeisberg M, Kalluri R. Physiology of the renal interstitium. Clin J Am Soc Nephrol. 2015. doi:10.2215/CJN.00640114. http://cjasn.asnjournals.org/content/early/2015/03/25/CJN.00640114.full.
2. Bernhardt WM, Wiesener MS, Scigalla P, Chou J, Schmieder RE, Günzler V, Eckardt K-U. Inhibition of prolyl hydroxylases increases erythropoietin production in ESRD. J Am Soc

Nephrol. 2010;21(12):2151–6. doi:10.1681/ASN.2010010116. http://www.ncbi.nlm.nih.gov/pmc/articles/PMC3014028/.

3. Teehan G, Benz RL. An update on the controversies in anemia management in chronic kidney disease: lessons learned and lost. Anemia. 2011;2011:623673. doi:10.1155/2011/623673. http://www.ncbi.nlm.nih.gov/pmc/articles/PMC3085324/.

4. Pham P-TT, Pham P-CT, Wilkinson AH, Lew SQ. Renal abnormalities in sickle cell disease. Kidney Int. 2000;57:1–8. doi:10.1046/j.1523-1755.2000.00806.x. http://www.nature.com/ki/journal/v57/n1/full/4491289a.html.

5. Nair RK, Khaira A, Sharma A, Mahajan S, Dinda AK. Spectrum of renal involvement in paroxysmal nocturnal hemoglobinuria: report of three cases and a brief review of the literature. Int Urol Nephrol. 2008;40(2):471–5. doi:10.1007/s11255-008-9356-5. http://link.springer.com/article/10.1007%2Fs11255-008-9356-5.

6. Noris M, Mescia F, Remuzzi G. STEC-HUS, atypical HUS and TTP are all diseases of complement activation. Nat Rev Nephrol. 2012;8:622–33. doi:10.1038/nrneph.2012.195. http://www.nature.com/nrneph/journal/v8/n11/full/nrneph.2012.195.html.

7. Dobre M, Rahman M, Hostetter TH. Current status of bicarbonate in CKD. J Am Soc Nephrol. 2015;26:515–23. doi:10.1681/ASN.2014020205. http://jasn.asnjournals.org/content/26/3/515.abstract.

8. de Brito-Ashurst I, Varagunam M, Raftery MJ, Yaqoob MM. Bicarbonate supplementation slows progression of CKD and improves nutritional status. J Am Soc Nephrol. 2009;20(9):2075. http://jasn.asnjournals.org/content/20/9/2075.full.pdf+html.

9. Goraya N, Simoni J, Jo C-H, Wesson DE. Treatment of metabolic acidosis in patients with stage 3 chronic kidney disease with fruits and vegetables or oral bicarbonate reduces urine angiotensinogen and preserves glomerular filtration rate. Kidney Int. 2014;86:1031–8. doi:10.1038/ki.2014.83. http://www.nature.com/ki/journal/v86/n5/full/ki201483a.html.

10. Saldana TM, Basso O, Darden R, Sandler DP. Carbonated beverages and chronic kidney disease. Epidemiology. 2007;18(4):501–6. http://www.ncbi.nlm.nih.gov/pmc/articles/PMC3433753/.

11. Al-Badr W, Martin KJ. Vitamin D and kidney disease. Clin J Am Soc Nephrol. 2008;3(5):1555–60. http://cjasn.asnjournals.org/content/3/5/1555.full.

12. Blaine J, Chonchol M, Levi M. Renal control of calcium, phosphate, and magnesium homeostasis. Clin J Am Soc Nephrol. 2015;10(7):1257–72. doi:10.2215/CJN.09750913. http://cjasn.asnjournals.org/content/10/7/1257.full.

13. Negri AL. Proximal tubule endocytic apparatus as the specific renal uptake mechanism for vitamin D-binding protein/25-(OH)D3 complex. Nephrology. 2006;11:510–5. http://onlinelibrary.wiley.com/enhanced/doi/10.1111/j.1440-1797.2006.00704.x/.

14. The EVOLVE Trial Investigators. Effect of cinacalcet on cardiovascular disease in patients undergoing dialysis. N Engl J Med. 2012;367:2482–94. doi:10.1056/NEJMoa1205624. http://www.nejm.org/doi/full/10.1056/NEJMoa1205624#t=articleTop.

15. Goldenstein PT, Elias RM, Pires de Freitas do Carmo L, Coelho FO, Magalhaes LP, et al. Parathyroidectomy improves survival in patients with severe hyperparathyroidism: a comparative study. PLoS One. 2013;8(8):e68870. doi:10.1371/journal.pone.0068870. http://journals.plos.org/plosone/article?id=10.1371/journal.pone.0068870.

16. Komaba H, Taniguchi M, Wada A, Iseki K, Tsubakihara Y, Fukagawa M. Parathyroidectomy and survival among Japanese hemodialysis patients with secondary hyperparathyroidism. Kidney Int. 2015;88(2):350–9. doi:10.1038/ki.2015.72. Epub 2015 Mar 18. http://www.nature.com/ki/journal/v88/n2/full/ki201572a.html.

17. Levi M, Ellis MA, Berl T. Control of renal hemodynamics and glomerular filtration rate in chronic hypercalcemia. Role of prostaglandins, renin-angiotensin system, and calcium. J Clin Invest. 1983;71(6):1624. http://dm5migu4zj3pb.cloudfront.net/manuscripts/110000/110918/JCI83110918.pdf.

Chapter 14
Immunology

Serological Tests That Help Diagnose Kidney Diseases

Abstract In this chapter we explain:

When immunology tests are most helpful
How diagnostic information is gained from measuring:

- Immunoglobulins and free light chains
- Anti-nuclear antibody
- Complement components C3 and C4
- Anti-neutrophil cytoplasmic antibody (ANCA)
- Anti-glomerular basement membrane antibody
- Anti-phospholipase A_2 receptor antibody

Do the Right Test on the Right Patient

The kidney is vulnerable to damage by the immune system [1]. The high blood flow rate through glomeruli exposes them to immunologically active cells. Antibodies and lymphocytes can attack vascular endothelial cells. Antigen-antibody complexes and complement molecules are trapped within the filtration barrier and taken up into mesangial cells and podocytes by endocytosis. Antibodies can be generated against antigens expressed in the glomerular basement membrane or on podocytes. Cell injury, inflammation and repair responses cause a wide range of kidney diseases.

Immunological tests on serum can help distinguish between conditions with clinically similar presentations. It is tempting to tick a number of boxes on the blood test request form to check for immune-mediated disease – a kidney disease 'immunology screen'. However, this may not be a wise move.

There is a danger of a false positive result with all screening tests. The likelihood that a positive result will be 'false' is dependent upon the pre-test probability – the prior odds – that the patient actually has the disease in question.

For example, the chances of an anti-nuclear antibody (ANA) test being positive in a healthy older person can be as high as one in five. The chances that someone with slowly progressive chronic kidney disease with minimal proteinuria has systemic lupus erythematosus (SLE) are perhaps one in a thousand. So a positive ANA test in such a person has a 1000/5 = 200 to 1 chance of being a false positive.

Similarly, serum IgA levels are elevated in a high proportion of patients with IgA nephropathy. A raised level can be useful supportive evidence in a patient with other typical features of IgA nephropathy. However, serum IgA is elevated in many other conditions including chronic infection and so on its own is not diagnostically specific [2].

The risk of ignoring these laws of probability is that you will be led along a path of ever-more invasive tests to exclude a serious cause for the abnormal result. For example, immunoglobulins and a protein electrophoresis are often assayed in patients with chronic kidney disease to 'exclude' multiple myeloma. The finding of a monoclonal paraprotein raises the possibility that the paraprotein is the cause of the kidney disease and the patient would benefit from chemotherapy. In reality, it is more likely that the paraprotein is unrelated to the kidney disease, a monoclonal protein of undetermined significance (MGUS). You may be left with the dilemma of whether to exclude monoclonal protein-related kidney disease by performing a renal biopsy.

The following sections describe the most commonly used immunological tests with the clinical features that indicate when they are likely to have diagnostic value.

Immunoglobulins, Protein Electrophoresis, Free Light Chains in Serum and Urine

Clinical features:

1. Multiple myeloma with myeloma kidney

   - Anaemia
   - Deteriorating GFR
   - Minimal proteinuria on dipstick testing but raised urine protein:creatinine ratio
   - Bone pain with normal alkaline phosphatase
   - Hypercalcaemia

2. Amyloidosis

   - Nephrotic-range proteinuria or nephrotic syndrome
   - Hypotension
   - Heart failure
   - Bruising

Free lights chains are smaller than albumin and freely filtered by glomeruli. Their serum concentration is therefore dependent upon GFR and patients with reduced GFR have increased serum levels of polyclonal free light chains. The levels are further increased by inflammation and are associated with an increased risk of progression of chronic kidney disease and of mortality [3].

The ratio of kappa to lambda light chain concentrations is used to identify a monoclonal excess of one type of chain. An abnormal ratio is not proof of clonality; further tests are needed to prove a monoclonal plasma cell disorder.

Monoclonal free light chains in the urine (Bence Jones protein) are not detected by dipstick testing but the laboratory urine protein assay does detect them. A specific test for free light chain is the most sensitive.

Multiple Myeloma

The kidneys can be damaged in patients with myeloma through a range of mechanisms. Hypercalcaemia has a direct effect on GFR (see Sect. "Hypercalcaemia" in page 189). Filtered free light chains are reabsorbed by proximal tubular cells and can cause cell injury. If light chains are in large amounts, they may combine with uromodulin to form casts that obstruct the tubules – 'cast nephropathy'.

It is helpful to compare changes over time in the amount of monoclonal protein in serum with the eGFR. If the two mirror each other, the monoclonal protein is more likely to be causing the decline in GFR and so be a monoclonal protein of renal significance (MGRS) rather than of undetermined significance (MGUS) [4] (Patient 14.1).

Patient 14.1: Myeloma Kidney
Mrs. Drake suffered repeated relapses of her myeloma over the course of four years, shown by rises in the concentration of monoclonal protein (Fig. 14.1).

During the first relapse in 2008 her kidney function was not affected.

During the second and third relapses in 2009 and 2010 her eGFR declined as the paraprotein level rose. Both times, further treatment led to a decline in paraprotein and recovery in eGFR.

Sadly her disease continued to progress and became unresponsive to treatment after 2010. She died in 2011.

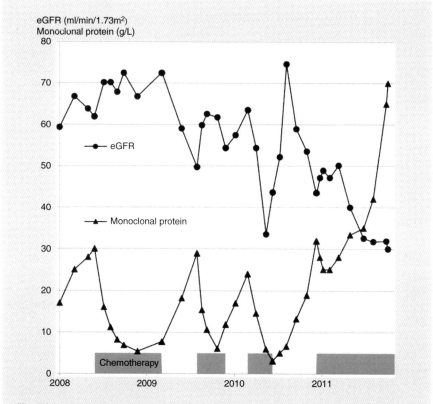

Fig. 14.1 eGFR mirrors the rises and falls in the concentration of monoclonal protein in a patient with multiple myeloma

Amyloidosis

Systemic amyloidosis refers to a group of conditions in which a small subunit of a plasma protein undergoes polymerisation and is deposited in the tissues as a fibril with a beta-pleated sheet configuration.

Examples of the proteins that can form amyloid deposits are:

- Immunoglobulin light chain (25 kDa): AL amyloidosis in plasma cell dyscrasia
- Serum amyloid A (12 kDa): AA amyloidosis in chronic inflammation
- Beta-2 microglobulin (12 kDa): Dialysis amyloidosis

The kidneys can be affected by deposition of amyloid protein into vessel walls and glomerular membranes (Figs. 14.2 and 14.3). This disrupts the filtration

Fig. 14.2 Light micrographs of a section of a renal biopsy from a patient with amyloidosis stained with Congo red. (**a**) Amyloid, coloured red, is deposited throughout the glomerulus and in the wall of an arteriole (*top left*). (**b**) anomalous colours are displayed when the specimen is examined between a crossed polarizer and analyser [5]. ×200

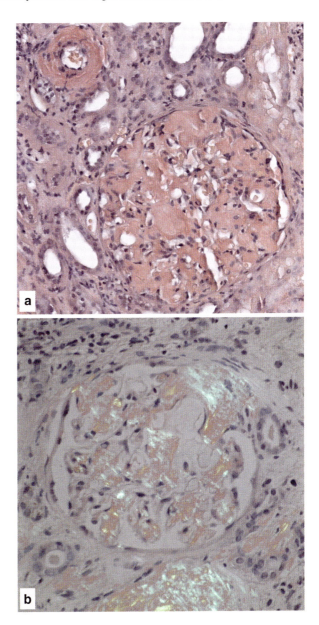

barrier allowing proteinuria that is often severe enough to cause the nephrotic syndrome.

Amyloid protein may also affect systemic arteriolar walls and the autonomic nerve fibres that mediate vasoconstriction. This causes postural hypotension and can reduce kidney blood flow.

Fig. 14.3 Electron micrograph showing amyloid fibrils (*star*) deposited in the glomerular basement membrane

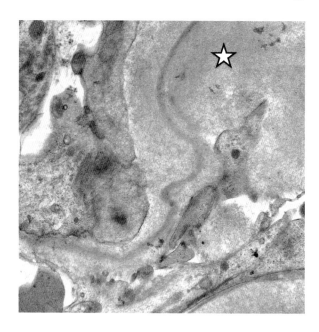

Anti-nuclear Antibody, Anti-dsDNA Antibody

Clinical features:
Systemic lupus erythematosus (SLE) nephritis

Nephritic syndrome:

- Proteinuria ++ or greater
- Microscopic ++ or greater
- Macroscopic haematuria (see Fig. 11.2)
- Worsening GFR over weeks or months

About half of people with SLE have kidney involvement, this proportion being higher in men and in black races. The pattern of kidney disease is very variable, ranging from asymptomatic urine abnormalities to acute nephritis and nephrotic syndrome. A biopsy is required to characterise the type of kidney disease.

Histological appearances are grouped into six classes, each associated with different clinical features and requiring different treatment [6].

Complement C3 and C4

Clinical features:
Glomerulonephritis

Nephritic syndrome:

- Proteinuria ++ or greater
- Microscopic ++ or greater
- Macroscopic haematuria (see Fig. 11.2)
- Worsening GFR over days, weeks or months

Components of the complement cascade (Fig. 14.4) are consumed in a range of auto-immune disorders.

Immune complexes of antibody and antigen are deposited in the glomeruli where they can fix complement and cause glomerulonephritis. Deposits of the C3 component of complement are the common feature in a recently characterised category of glomerulonephritis [7].

Serum C3 and C4 levels are reduced in patients with nephritis associated with SLE and cryoglobulinaemia. This suggests activation of the classical and alternative pathways. C4 levels may be unreliable for monitoring SLE nephritis because genetic deficiencies of C4 are relatively common and cause a low C4 without disease.

C3 is usually decreased more than C4 in patients with C3 glomerulopathy, Dense Deposit Disease, post-streptococcal glomerulonephritis, bacterial endocarditis glomerulonephritis and cholesterol crystal embolism. This suggests activation of the alternative pathway.

The drop in C3 found in children with post-streptococcal glomerulonephritis is usually short lasting. If the level of C3 remains low for longer than eight weeks, the autoantibody 'C3 nephritic factor' that blocks the regulation of C3 activation may be present [8].

Fig. 14.4 The main elements of the complement cascade. Immune complexes activate the classical pathway, lowering levels of both C3 and C4. When the alternative pathway is activated, typically C3 is low but C4 is normal. Factor H and CD46 inhibit the alternative pathway C3 convertase. If they are defective, the alternative pathway is overactive and leads to cell damage by the generation of membrane attack complexes (C5b-9). Eculizumab blocks C5 cleavage and is used to control overactivity of the alternative pathway in atypical haemolytic uraemic syndrome (aHUS) (see Sect. "Kidney disease linked to causes of anaemia" in page 176)

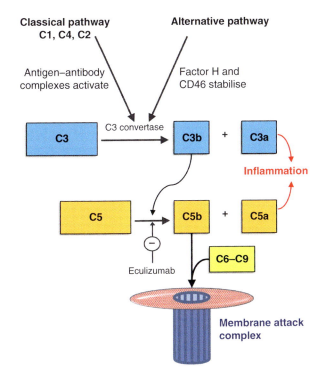

Anti-streptolysin O (ASO) and Anti-DNAse B Antibodies

Clinical features:
Post-streptococcal glomerulonephritis

Nephritic syndrome:

- Oedema and hypertension
- Proteinuria ++ or greater
- Microscopic ++ or greater
- Macroscopic haematuria (see Fig. 11.2)
- Worsening GFR over days

Although rare in industrialized countries, in the developing world there are between 10 and 30 cases of post-streptococcal glomerulonephritis per 100,000 people per year. It typically follows a streptococcal sore throat in children and the skin infection impetigo in older adults with comorbidities. Antibodies are generated in response to infections with Group A and sometimes Group C Streptococci. C3 levels are low because the alternative pathway of complement is activated (see Fig. 14.4).

The onset of nephritis with smoky brown-red haematuria (see Fig. 11.2) is classically two weeks after the onset of the infection, in contrast to the haematuria that occurs at the time of the sore throat in IgA nephropathy. Streptococcal antigens are deposited between the basement membrane and podocytes where they form immune complexes with antibodies. These stimulate an influx of acute inflammatory cells – a proliferative glomerulonephritis (Fig. 14.5).

As well as anti-streptolysin O (ASO) antibodies, anti-hyaluronidase (AHase), anti-streptokinase (ASKase), anti-nicotinamide-adenine dinucleotidase (anti-NAD) and anti-DNAse B antibodies may be detected. ASO, anti-DNAse B, anti-NAD, and AHase titers are commonly elevated after a pharyngeal infection. Only the anti-DNAse B and AHase titers are typically increased after a skin infection. The rise in ASO titre may be blunted by antibiotic therapy.

The prognosis varies with age; in children kidney function usually returns to normal whereas the elderly may have persistent chronic kidney disease and a mortality rate of up to 25 % [9].

Anti-neutrophil Cytoplasmic Antibody (ANCA)

- Cytoplasmic or C-ANCA
- Perinuclear or P-ANCA, either typical or atypical
- Anti-myeloperoxidase (MPO)
- Anti-proteinase 3 (PR3)

Clinical features:
Systemic vasculitis with glomerulonephritis

- PR3-ANCA (usually C-ANCA) is associated with Granulomatosis with Polyangiitis (GPA, formerly Wegener's granulomatosis)

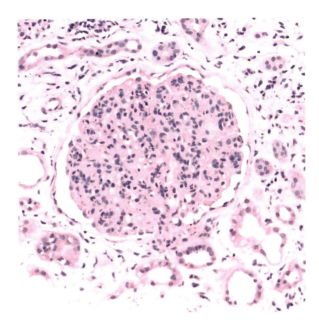

Fig. 14.5 Section of a renal biopsy from a patient with nephritis following a streptococcal sore throat. There is global endocapillary hypercellularity with infiltration of neutrophils and mononuclear cells and obliteration of the peripheral glomerular capillary loops. This glomerulus is representative of all in the specimen, i.e. the glomerulonephritis is diffuse and proliferative

- MPO-ANCA (usually P-ANCA) is associated with Microscopic Polyangiitis (MPA) and Eosinophilic GPA (EGPA, formerly Churg-Strauss syndrome)
- Atypical-ANCA (negative for MPO and PR3 antibodies) occurs in many inflammatory conditions including inflammatory bowel disease and rheumatoid arthritis, and in some infections.

Vasculitic illness lasting a few weeks:

- Fevers, malaise, weight loss
- Arthralgia, purpuric rash
- ENT symptoms, haemoptysis,
- Uveitis
- Mononeuritis multiplex

Nephritic syndrome:

- Proteinuria ++ or greater
- Microscopic ++ or greater
- Macroscopic haematuria (see Fig. 11.2)
- Worsening GFR over days or weeks

Patients with ANCA-associated vasculitis may have one or more features of a vasculitic illness in different combinations, giving rise to different disease subtypes. The diseases also tend to relapse and remit over time.

Serum is tested for ANCA by immunofluorescence, and for anti-PR3 and anti-MPO by enzyme-linked immunosorbent assay (ELISA). The results of the ELISA test are quantitative and more specific for different disease subtypes.

Fig. 14.6 Vasculitis with fibrinoid necrosis of a renal artery. There is destruction of the vessel wall which is replaced by *pink* fibrin. Mixed inflammatory cells surround and focally infiltrate the vessel wall. Haematoxylin and eosin ×200

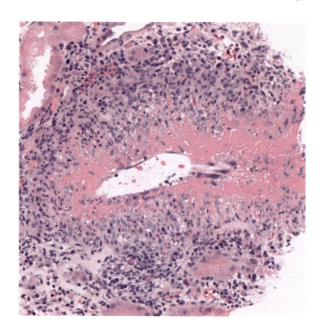

ANCA antibodies bind to antigens in neutrophils and monocytes [10]. The cells are activated and cluster at sites of inflammation where they release webs of fibres called Neutrophil Extracellular Traps (NETs) which normally capture and kill micro-organisms. The cells damage the endothelium of blood vessels and cause fibrinoid necrosis (Fig. 14.6) [11].

Patient 14.2: ANCA Positive, Anti-PR3 Positive Vasculitis

Mr. Grantham, a 70-year-old retired businessman, became increasingly unwell over a few months with lethargy, fever, joint pains, weight loss and painful numbness in his feet. There was blood +++ and protein +++ on the urine dipstick test. His eGFR fell from 70 to 30 over 1 week.

His C-reactive protein (CRP) was high (99 mg/L). The ANCA test was positive with a cytoplasmic pattern (c-ANCA). Proteinase 3 (PR3) antibodies were present at 91 IU/ml (normal range 0.2–1.9). Myeloperoxidase (MPO) antibodies were not increased (0.2 IU/ml, NR 0.2–3.4).

A kidney biopsy showed a focal segmental glomerulonephritis with necrosis and crescents (Fig. 14.7). There was no significant deposition of immunoglobulins or complement, consistent with a pauci-immune glomerulonephritis.

He was treated with intravenous methylprednisolone followed by daily oral prednisolone and three-weekly doses of intravenous cyclophosphamide. His symptoms settled and the PR3 antibody titre and CRP fell quickly. His eGFR rose over the following five months (Fig. 14.8). He was left with some distressing painful neuropathy in his feet.

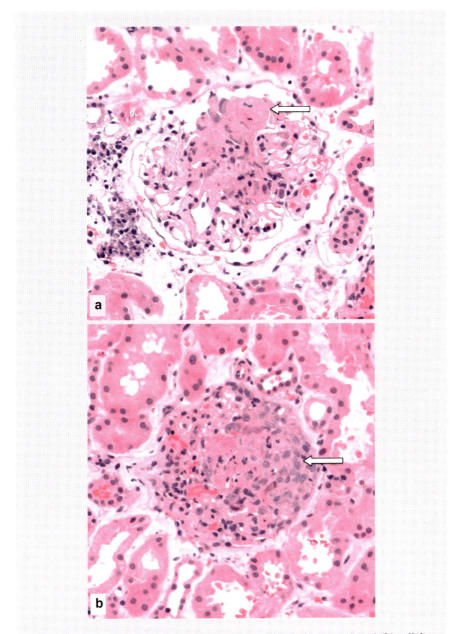

Fig. 14.7 Glomeruli showing (**a**) segmental necrotising lesion (*arrow*) and (**b**) cellular crescent (*arrow*). Haematoxylin and eosin ×200

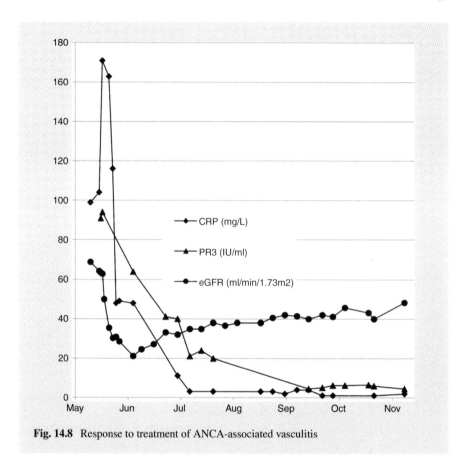

Fig. 14.8 Response to treatment of ANCA-associated vasculitis

Not all ANCA antibodies are pathogenic. Some are non-specific markers of inflammatory disease and their presence does not necessarily mean that the kidneys are involved in a vasculitic illness.

In someone with systemic vasculitis, the titre of an ANCA antibody is not a direct measure of disease activity. A rising titre does indicate an increased risk of relapse of the kidney disease but should not be used to guide immunosuppressive treatment. Less than half of patients with a rising titre suffer a clinical relapse within the next year. On the other hand, a negative ANCA is reassuring as the risk of relapse is very low [12].

If someone has a past history of vasculitis and the immunosuppression has been reduced or stopped, it is helpful to compare any new symptoms with the original vasculitic illness to decide if the disease has come back (Patient 14.3).

Patient 14.3: ANCA Positive, Anti-MPO Positive Vasculitis

Mr. Austin had been taking prednisolone and azathioprine for microscopic polyangiitis for many years. In 2012, routine monitoring of the anti-MPO titre showed a sudden increase associated with a modest rise in CRP but no drop in eGFR (Fig. 14.9).

Although he felt well, a thorough search for disease activity revealed a new nodule in the lung on a CT scan. The dose of prednisolone was increased for 3 months.

Two years later the anti-MPO titre steadily increased but he remained completely well, with no change in CRP or eGFR and no proteinuria. Treatment was not increased but he was monitored closely for symptoms of disease activity.

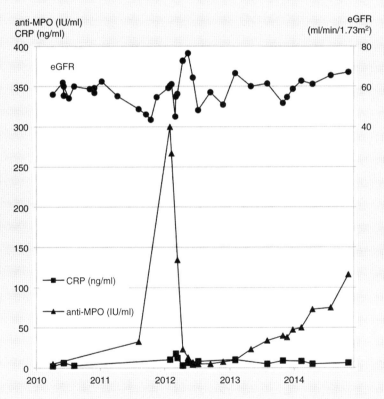

Fig. 14.9 Periods of acute and progressive increase in the titre of anti-MPO antibody that were not associated with a decline in eGFR

Anti-glomerular Basement Membrane Antibody (Anti-GBM ab)

Clinical features:
Anti-GBM disease (Goodpasture's syndrome)

Acute nephritic syndrome:

- Proteinuria ++ or greater
- Microscopic ++ or greater
- Macroscopic haematuria (see Fig. 11.2)
- Worsening GFR over days

Alveolar haemorrhage with haemoptysis

Patients with anti-GBM disease are usually very ill. The diagnosis should be confirmed urgently by testing serum for anti-GBM antibodies and, if there is any doubt about the diagnosis, by kidney biopsy (Fig. 14.10). Intensive immunosuppressive therapy including plasma exchange is indicated for kidney disease and lung haemorrhage.

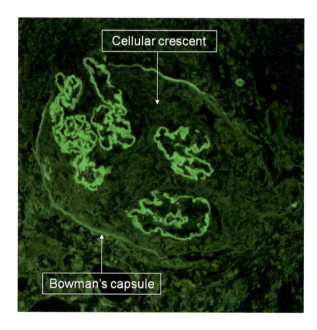

Fig. 14.10 Glomerulus stained with fluorescent-labelled anti-IgG from a patient with anti-GBM disease. The continuous linear staining indicates that IgG antibody has bound all along the glomerular basement membrane. Bowman's space around the glomerular tuft is filled with a crescent (Image provided by Professor Agnes Fogo)

Anti-phospholipase A$_2$ Receptor Antibody (Anti-PLA$_2$R ab)

Clinical features:
Membranous glomerulonephritis (MN)

Nephrotic-range proteinuria or nephrotic syndrome, in adults

The majority of patients with MN have circulating autoantibodies against the M-type phospholipase A$_2$ receptor (PLA$_2$R) which is located on normal podoctyes [13]. The function of the PLA$_2$R is unknown. The protein was named according to the location of its gene but in humans it does not actually bind PLA$_2$.

A positive anti-PLA$_2$R antibody test is increasingly accepted as diagnostic of idiopathic MN in adults with nephrotic syndrome who do not have signs of a primary cause. It may avoid the need for a renal biopsy in such patients [14].

Antibody levels parallel changes in the level of proteinuria and help predict the response to treatment and the risk of relapse of nephrotic syndrome.

Some patients with idiopathic MN without anti-PLA$_2$R antibodies have circulating autoantibodies against thrombospondin type-1 domain-containing 7A (THSD7A) [15].

Immune complexes of PLA$_2$R antigen and IgG$_4$ are formed in the space between the glomerular basement membrane and the podocytes. Their presence stimulates the membrane to thicken around them (Fig. 14.11) forming 'spikes' seen by light microscopy with a silver stain (Fig. 14.12) and electron microscopy (Fig. 14.13).

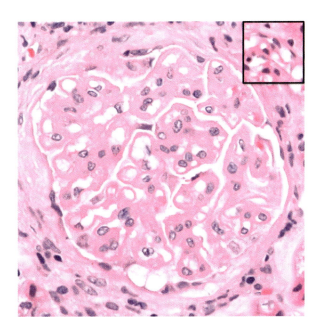

Fig. 14.11 Glomerulus affected by membranous nephropathy. Glomerular capillary membranes are thickened (haematoxylin and eosin ×400). The *inset* shows the thickness of normal membranes for comparison

Fig. 14.12 External
surfaces of the capillary
loops have spikes
protruding from them. The
spikes are separated by
spaces containing immune
deposits that do not take up
the silver stain. Some
sections of the glomerular
basement membrane are
thickened and contain
holes where deposits have
been enclosed within the
membrane (*inset*) (silver
×400)

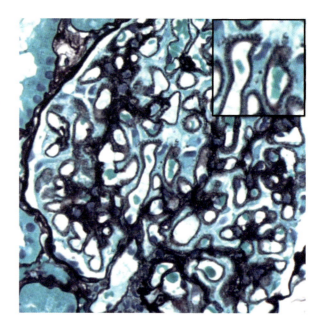

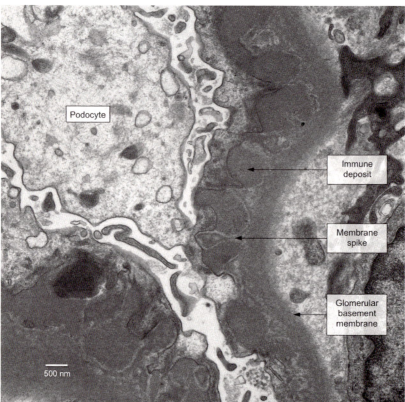

Fig. 14.13 Subepithelial immune deposits between the glomerular basement membrane and a podocyte with spikes of membrane between adjacent deposits (EM ×13,000)

References

1. Yatim KM, Lakkis FG. A brief journey through the immune system. Clin J Am Soc Nephrol. 2015;10(7):1274–81. doi:10.2215/CJN.10031014. http://cjasn.asnjournals.org/content/early/2015/04/06/CJN.10031014.full.
2. J Maeda A, Gohda T, Funabiki K, Horikoshi S, Shirato I, Tomino Y. Significance of serum IgA levels and serum IgA/C3 ratio in diagnostic analysis of patients with IgA nephropathy. Clin Lab Anal. 2003;17(3):73–6. http://onlinelibrary.wiley.com/doi/10.1002/jcla.10071/abstract;jsessionid=A271E49EC0DF8F1FF6196265F755FA83.f02t02.
3. Ritchie J, Assi LK, Burmeister A, Hoefield R, Cockwell P, Kalra PA. Association of serum Ig free light chains with mortality and ESRD among patients with nondialysis-dependent CKD. Clin J Am Soc Nephrol. 2015;10(5):740–9. doi:10.2215/CJN.09660914. http://cjasn.asnjournals.org/content/early/2015/03/30/CJN.09660914.
4. Leung N, Bridoux F, Hutchison CA, Nasr SH, Cockwell P, Fermand J-P, Dispenzieri A, Song KW, Kyle RA. Monoclonal gammopathy of renal significance: when MGUS is no longer undetermined or insignificant. Blood. 2012;120(22):4292–5. doi:10.1182/blood-2012-07-445304. http://www.bloodjournal.org/content/120/22/4292.long?sso-checked=true.
5. Howie AJ, Brewer DB, Howell D, Jones AP. Physical basis of colors seen in Congo red-stained amyloid in polarized light. Lab Invest. 2008;88(3):232–42. doi:10.1038/labinvest.3700714. Epub 2007 Dec 31. http://www.nature.com/labinvest/journal/v88/n3/full/3700714a.html.
6. Hahn BH, McMahon MA, Wilkinson A, Wallace WD, Daikh DI, Fitzgerald JD, Karpouzas GA, Merrill JT, Wallace DJ, Yazdany J, Ramsey-Goldman R, Singh K, Khalighi M, Choi SI, Gogia M, Kafaja S, Kamgar M, Lau C, Martin WJ, Parikh S, Peng J, Rastogi A, Chen W, Grossman JM, American College of Rheumatology. American College of Rheumatology guidelines for screening, treatment, and management of lupus nephritis. Arthritis Care Res (Hoboken). 2012;64(6):797–808. doi:10.1002/acr.21664. http://www.ncbi.nlm.nih.gov/pmc/articles/PMC3437757/.
7. Fakhouri F, Frémeaux-Bacchi V, Noël LH, Cook HT, Pickering MC. C3 glomerulopathy: a new classification. Nat Rev Nephrol. 2010;6(8):494–9. doi:10.1038/nrneph.2010.85. http://www.nature.com/nrneph/journal/v6/n8/full/nrneph.2010.85.html.
8. Paixão-Cavalcante D, López-Trascasa M, Skattum L, Giclas PC, Goodship TH, Rodríguez de Córdoba S, Truedsson L, Morgan BP, Harris CL. Sensitive and specific assays for C3 nephritic factors clarify mechanisms underlying complement dysregulation. Kidney Int. 2012;82:1084–92. doi:10.1038/ki.2012.250. http://www.nature.com/ki/journal/v82/n10/full/ki2012250a.html.
9. Rodriguez-Iturbe B, Musser JM. The current state of poststreptococcal glomerulonephritis. J Am Soc Nephrol. 2008;19:1855–64. doi:10.1681/ASN.2008010092. http://jasn.asnjournals.org/content/19/10/1855.full.
10. Jennette JC, Falk RJ. ANCAs are also antimonocyte cytoplasmic autoantibodies. Clin J Am Soc Nephrol. 2015;10(1):4–6. doi:10.2215/CJN.11501114. http://cjasn.asnjournals.org/content/10/1/4.short.
11. Schoenermarck U, Csernok E, Gross WL. Pathogenesis of anti-neutrophil cytoplasmic antibody-associated vasculitis: challenges and solutions 2014. Nephrol Dial Transplant. 2015;30 Suppl 1:i46–52. doi:10.1093/ndt/gfu398. http://ndt.oxfordjournals.org/content/30/suppl_1/i46.abstract.
12. Kemna MJ, Damoiseaux J, Austen J, Winkens B, Peters J, van Paassen P, Tervaert JWC. ANCA as a predictor of relapse: useful in patients with renal involvement but not in patients with nonrenal disease. J Am Soc Nephrol. 2015;26:537–42. doi:10.1681/ASN.2013111233. http://jasn.asnjournals.org/content/26/3/537.abstract.
13. Stehlé T, Audard V, Ronco P, Debiec H. Phospholipase A2 receptor and sarcoidosis-associated membranous nephropathy. Nephrol Dial Transplant. 2015;30(6):1047–50. doi:10.1093/ndt/gfv080. http://ndt.oxfordjournals.org/content/early/2015/04/02/ndt.gfv080.short?rss=1.
14. Hofstra JM, Wetzels JFM. Phospholipase A2 receptor antibodies in membranous nephropathy: unresolved issues. J Am Soc Nephrol. 2014;25:1137–9. doi:10.1681/ASN.2014010091. http://jasn.asnjournals.org/content/25/6/1137.long.

15. Tomas NM, Beck LH, Meyer-Schwesinger C, Seitz-Polski B, Ma H, Zahner G, Dolla G, Hoxha E, Helmchen U, Dabert-Gay A-S, Debayle D, Merchant M, Klein J, Salant DJ, Stahl RAK, Lambeau G. Thrombospondin type-1 domain-containing 7A in idiopathic membranous nephropathy. N Engl J Med. 2014;371:2277–87. doi:10.1056/NEJMoa1409354. http://www. nejm.org/doi/pdf/10.1056/NEJMoa1409354.

Chapter 15
Image the Urinary Tract

Strengths and Weaknesses of Different Radiology Modalities

Abstract In this chapter we explain:

- The common abnormalities found by ultrasound scanning the urinary tract
- How urinary tract obstruction is investigated
- How radio-isotope scanning measures kidney perfusion and excretion
- How CT scanning is used to diagnose kidney stones
- The risks and benefits of using radio-contrast

Ultrasound

The most common modality for imaging the urinary tract is plain ultrasound (Figs. 15.1 and 15.2).

Appearances in Kidney Disease

Changes to the ultrasound appearance are seen in both acute and chronic kidney disease. Cellular infiltration, interstitial oedema, sclerosis of glomeruli and fibrosis all non-specifically increase the reflectivity to ultrasound, or 'brightness', of the image. This is most easily judged by comparing the reflectivity of the renal cortex with the adjacent liver. The scan report may describe 'increased cortical echo-genicity' and/or 'loss of cortico-medullary differentiation'.

The kidney may shrink in volume as chronic damage progresses and ultimately it can be hard to distinguish the kidney from the surrounding tissues (Fig. 15.3). Localised damage and scarring may make the outline of the kidney irregular (Fig. 15.4).

Cysts are a frequent incidental finding and may cause concern to the patient and doctor (Fig. 15.5). They may be multiple, large and in both kidneys (see Sect. "Cystic kidney diseases" in page 91). Patients with end-stage kidney disease often

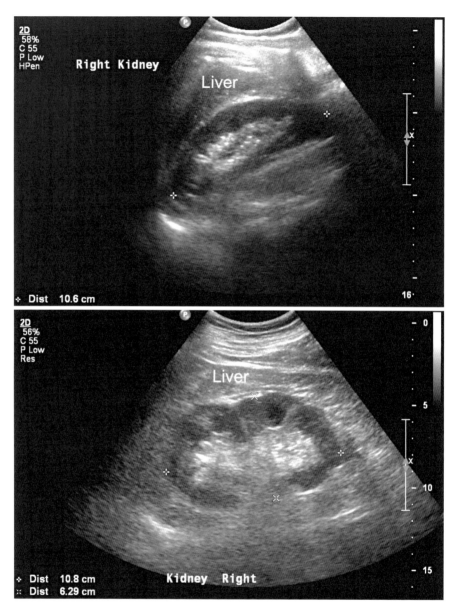

Figs. 15.1 and 15.2 Ultrasound scans of normal kidneys. The renal cortex is of the same or lower echogenicity (reflectivity) than the liver or spleen. The liver lies immediately superior to the right kidney. The centrally placed renal sinus fat is of greater echogenicity than both the renal cortex and the liver and spleen

develop cysts in their small kidneys – acquired cystic disease – which uncommonly can progress to carcinoma.

Cysts are classified according to the presence of internal membranes (septa), calcification and solid structures within them – the Bosniak classification [1]. If the cysts have a thin wall and do not contain septa, calcification or solid structures, they

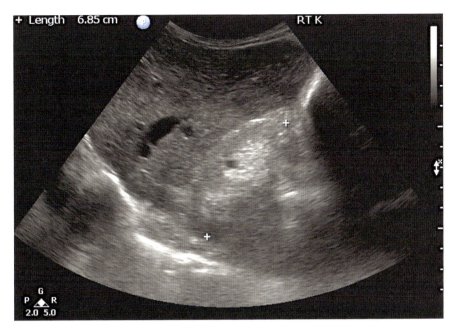

Fig. 15.3 Ultrasound scan of a small (6.85 cm in length) chronically damaged right kidney. The cortex is thinned and appears brighter than the liver, which lies above it. Both cortex and medulla are hyperechoic, obliterating the normal differentiation between them

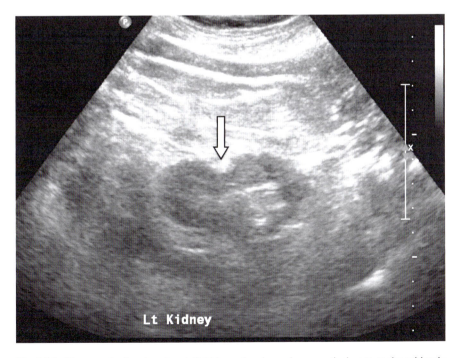

Fig. 15.4 Ultrasound of a shrunken left kidney showing a large cortical scar at the mid-pole (*arrow*)

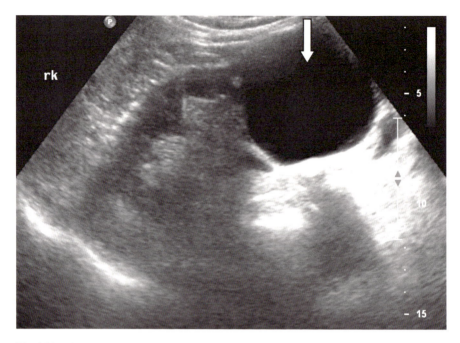

Fig. 15.5 Ultrasound scan of a right kidney containing a simple thin walled cyst on the lower pole, 6.2 cm in diameter (*arrow*). Otherwise the kidney is normal in appearance

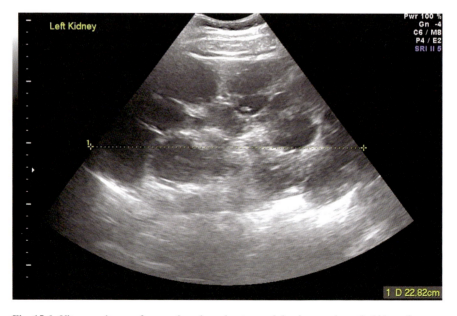

Fig. 15.6 Ultrasound scan of a grossly enlarged autosomal dominant polycystic kidney that was easily felt on physical examination

Figs. 15.7, 15.8 and 15.9 Ultrasound scans of the right and left kidneys and bladder in a patient with chronic bladder outflow obstruction. Both kidneys show gross hydronephrosis. The bladder is distended and the wall is thickened (1.84 cm) with an irregular trabeculated surface. In a man, these appearances are usually caused by prostatic enlargement. These images are from a woman with a urethral stricture

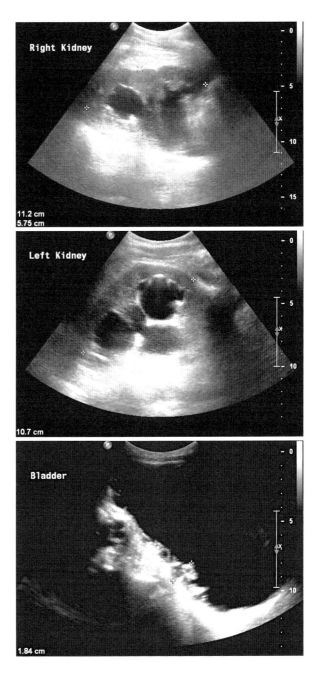

are benign and of no clinical significance. In particular, they do not cause pain unless they become infected or there is bleeding into them.

In autosomal dominant polycystic kidney disease in adults the cysts are more numerous, the kidneys become enlarged and the remaining tissues are distorted (Fig. 15.6). Cysts may also be found in the liver and spleen.

Urinary Tract Obstruction

Ultrasound is the first modality to use for detecting obstruction to urinary flow at any level of the urinary tract. In a hydronephrotic kidney, dilation of the renal sinuses and calyces is seen as a branching fluid space within the echogenic central sinus area (Figs. 15.7, 15.8 and 15.9). Occasionally, centrally placed cysts can mimic this appearance.

If the obstruction occurred very recently the kidney may appear entirely normal on ultrasound, with no visible hydronephrosis. If a patient has clinical features that suggest obstruction, even a suggestion of dilatation of the collecting system should prompt further studies (Patient 15.1).

Patient 15.1: Retroperitoneal Fibrosis
Mr. Castle, aged 60, went to donate blood and was found to be anaemic, Hb = 108 g/L. He had been tired over the previous 3 weeks but apart from some back pain had no other symptoms. As part of further investigation his eGFR was found to be 11 ml/min/1.73 m^2 so he was referred to hospital urgently. He had no past or family history of kidney disease but was hypertensive, BP = 196/119 mmHg. His ECG showed left ventricular hypertrophy. Urine albumin:creatinine ratio was normal, 1.8 mg/mmol (15.8 mg/g). CRP was raised, 71 mg/L.

The report on an urinary tract ultrasound scan (Figs. 15.10 and 15.11) stated: "minimal fullness of the collecting system is noted bilaterally, otherwise both kidneys appear normal in size and echopattern. Renal lengths were: Right 10.7 cm, Left 10.4 cm. No scarring or obvious renal calculi seen."

Doppler ultrasound studies showed normal kidney blood flow but there was considerable atheroma lining the anterior wall of the aorta, measuring 1.27 cm in AP depth (Fig. 15.12).

The medical team interpreted the ultrasound scan report as indicating that there was no obstruction and he was referred to the renal medicine team. They reviewed the images and suspecting bilateral hydronephrosis they obtained a second opinion. This confirmed hydronephrosis and bilateral nephrostomies were inserted.

Nephrostogram studies showed dilated pelvicalyceal systems in both kidneys with medial deviation and narrowing of both ureters from L4 inferiorly (Fig. 15.13). This suggested bilateral extrinsic compression due to retroperitoneal fibrosis.

Stents were passed down the ureters via the nephrostomies and Mr. Castle's kidney function returned to normal over the following 6 weeks.

A CT urogram showed soft tissue around the aorta attached to the ureters, extending down to the common iliac arteries (Fig. 15.14).

These appearances are typical of retroperitoneal fibrosis, which is an inflammatory reaction to atheromatous material that has leaked out from the aorta into the surrounding retroperitoneal space [2].

He was treated with prednisolone and his back pain improved. The CRP returned to normal, 6 mg/L, and his anaemia resolved, Hb 141 g/L. A subsequent CT scan confirmed that the tissue had reduced in volume.

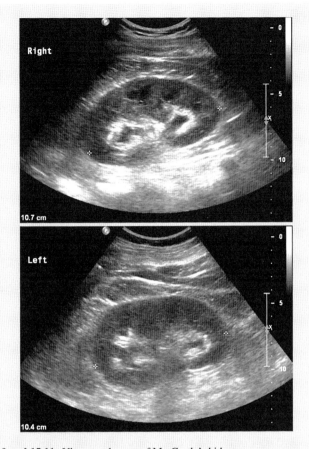

Figs. 15.10 and 15.11 Ultrasound scans of Mr. Castle's kidneys

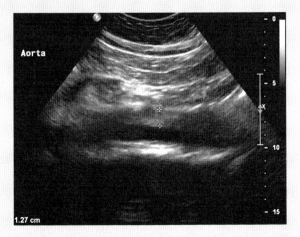

Fig. 15.12 Ultrasound scan of Mr. Castle's aorta

Fig. 15.13 Antegrade nephrostogram study showing dilated pelvicalyceal systems in both kidneys. The lower ureters are deviated medially and compressed by retroperitoneal fibrotic tissue

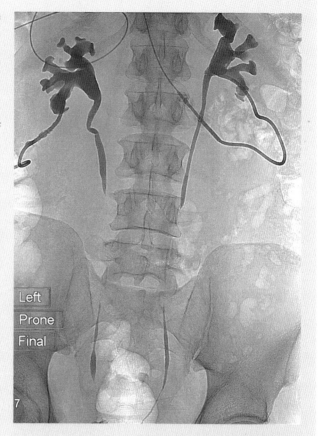

Fig. 15.14 CT urogram showing soft tissue around the aorta attached to the ureters that are identified by the radio-opaque stents within them

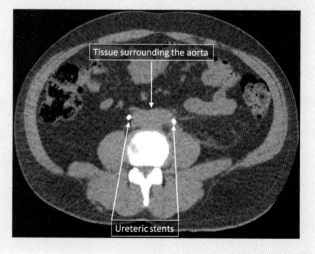

Dilatation of the collecting system in a kidney does not necessarily mean that it is obstructed. In the last trimester of pregnancy, normal kidneys can appear moderately hydronephrotic due to the pressure of the uterus and the effects of progesterone. A transplanted kidney usually has a dilated intrarenal collecting system. If there is doubt, a different type of scan is required that shows the flow of urine (see Sect. "Isotope renography" below).

Isotope Renography

There are two types of isotope kidney scan – static and dynamic. Static scans are taken to show the size of the kidneys and how evenly the isotope is distributed. An isotope is used that is concentrated and retained in the kidney, technetium 99 m dimercaptosuccinic acid (DMSA). If there is an area of scarring in one kidney or failure of the kidney to develop (renal agenesis), the isotope is not taken up. The DMSA scan is also the reference technique for showing the relative function between the two kidneys (see Patient 7.2).

A dynamic scan follows the flow of isotope in blood into the kidneys and out of them in urine. The patient receives an intravenous dose of the radioisotope technetium-99 m mercaptoacetyltriglycine (MAG3) that is concentrated in the kidneys and excreted in the urine. The trace of radioactivity is called a MAG3 renogram (see Patient 7.2). The MAG3 can be used like DMSA to produce a static scan (Figs. 15.15 and 15.16).

Radioactivity is counted to track the flow of isotope in urine out of the kidney (Fig. 15.17). Intravenous diuretic, furosemide, is given to maximise the flow of urine and accentuate any obstruction (Fig. 15.18).

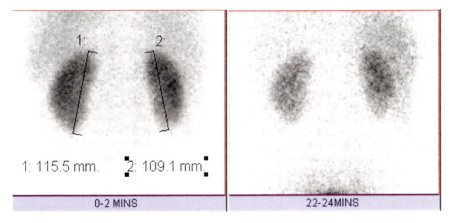

1: 115.5 mm.   2: 109.1 mm.

| 0-2 MINS | 22-24MINS |

Fig. 15.15 Static scans from a normal 99 m Tc MAG3 renogram. The kidneys are of normal size and shape: *left* (*1*) = 115.5 mm, *right* (*2*) 109.1 mm. The isotope is homogeneously distributed on the scan taken during the first 2 min. The level of radioactivity has declined symmetrically on the scan taken between 22 and 24 min

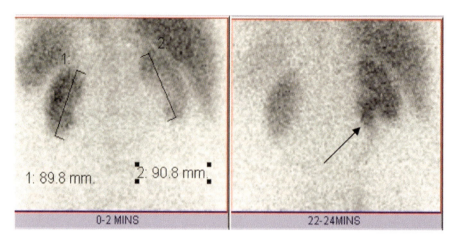

Fig. 15.16 A 99 m Tc MAG3 renogram with intravenous furosemide in a patient with a right hydronephrosis and hydroureter on an ultrasound scan. Both kidneys have cortical thinning and are smaller than normal: *left* (*1*) = 89.8 mm, *right* (*2*) = 90.8 mm; c.f. Fig. 15.15) but maintain a normal shape. On the scan taken in the first 2 min there is less uptake of isotope on the *right* (*2*) than the *left* (*1*). On the 22–24 min scan there is increased activity in the right pelvicalyceal system in keeping with ureteric obstruction (*arrow*)

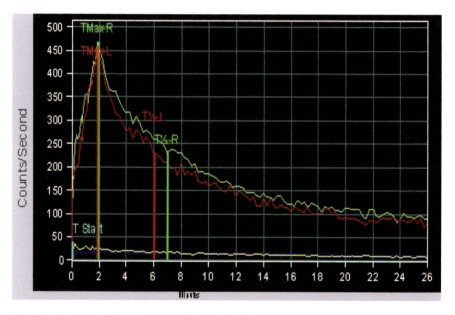

Fig. 15.17 A normal MAG3 renogram. There is rapid symmetrical uptake (TMax = 2 min, normal <6 min) and excretion of the isotope (T½ *left* = 6 min, T½ *right* = 7 min, normal <15 min)

The anatomical site of the obstruction is identified using an X-ray contrast study (Fig 15.19).

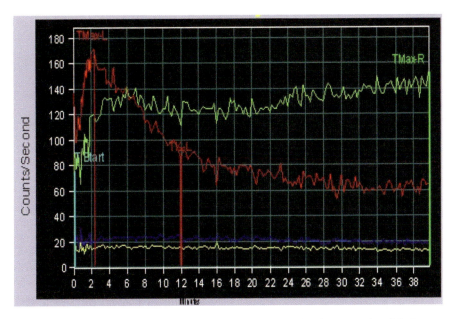

Fig. 15.18 MAG3 renogram in a patient with right hydroureter. Maximum uptake of the isotope is reduced in both kidneys compared to the normal scan (see Fig. 15.17) due to reduced GFR (TMax *left* = 170 counts/s, *right* = 150, normal = 450). The left kidney excretion curve (*TMaxL and T½ L in red*) is within normal limits (T½ = 12 min, normal <15 min). The right kidney curve (*TMax-R in yellow*) shows slower uptake and no decline, indicating obstruction to urinary flow

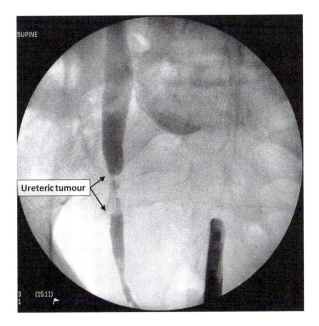

Fig. 15.19 Retrograde urogram shows a filling defect in the right ureter due to a ureteric tumour that is causing hydroureter, i.e. dilatation of the ureter above it

Computed Tomography

When imaging a patient who presents with suspected renal colic, it is common practice to perform a CT urogram rather than an ultrasound scan (Figs. 15.20 and 15.21). CT is more sensitive for calculi and allows other organs and blood vessels to be assessed on the same scan, theoretically increasing the diagnostic yield. However, if

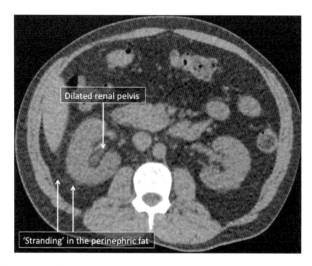

Fig. 15.20 Non-contrast CT scan showing hydronephrosis of the right kidney with 'stranding' due to increased pressure in the collecting system causing leakage of fluid into the fat around the kidney

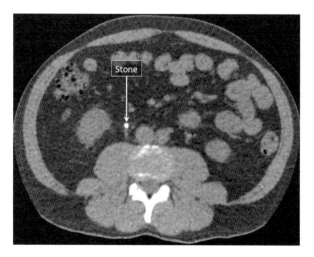

Fig. 15.21 CT scan section through the stone lodged in the ureter

Fig. 15.22 CT scan showing gas within the collecting system of an enlarged left kidney in a patient with emphysematous pyelonephritis

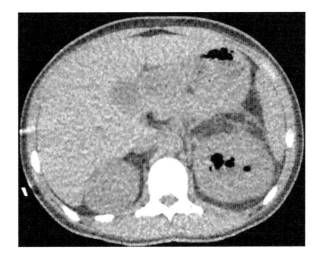

skilled ultrasound scanning is immediately available the superiority of CT has been questioned [3].

On a plain X-ray, stones vary in their opacity to the X-rays. Stones containing calcium (calcium oxalate, calcium phosphate) or struvite (magnesium ammonium phosphate) are opaque. Stones containing sulphur (cystine) are semi-opaque. Stones composed of uric acid, xanthine and pure matrix (coagulated mucoid material) are radiolucent [4].

No contrast is required with a CT scan because even radiolucent stones are visible, apart from the very rare pure matrix stones. This avoids any risk of contrast-induced nephropathy (see Sect. "The risks and benefits of using contrast media" below).

In patients with macroscopic haematuria but no colic, a soft tissue lesion is much more likely than a stone and so contrast is required.

CT is also good for visualising gas within and around the urinary tract. Gas can be produced in the urine of patients with diabetes from the fermentation of glucose by bacteria, usually *Eschericia coli* or *Klebsiella pneumoniae*. This causes a severe form of kidney infection – emphysematous pyelonephritis (Fig. 15.22) [5].

The Risks and Benefits of Using Contrast Media

To increase the differentiation between structures on an X-ray, radio-contrast medium is injected intravenously. The iodine in the medium attenuates the X-rays and creates a contrast in density between blood vessels and tissues with high and low blood flows (Figs. 15.23 and 15.24).

Media vary in their iodine content and this affects their osmolality; high-osmolar media have a higher ratio of iodine atoms to dissolved particles.

Patients with risk factors for acute kidney injury such as chronic kidney disease, diabetes mellitus, congestive heart failure, and older age are at risk of contrast-induced

Fig. 15.23 Normal CT urogram with contrast, highlighting the arterial blood supply to the kidneys

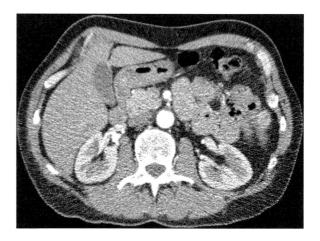

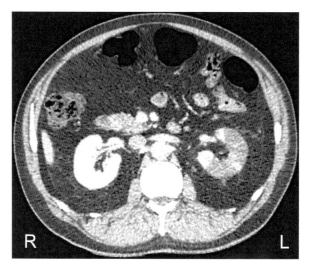

Fig. 15.24 CT urogram with contrast from a patient with chronic atrial fibrillation who suddenly developed severe left loin pain. There are segmental areas of low attenuation throughout the left kidney due to infarcts caused by emboli

nephropathy (CIN, or CI-AKI). It is another example of a MINT cocktail (see Sect. "Mixing vasoactive drugs to make MINT cocktails" in page 108) [6]. The injury is caused by vasoconstriction in the outer medulla of the kidney. This region normally has a limited blood supply so as not to wash away the urea concentration gradient. It is therefore vulnerable to ischaemic damage. Contrast agents may also have direct toxic effects on renal tubular cells.

The risk of CIN is greater with increasing volumes of contrast medium and with high- rather than low-osmolar contrast medium. Intravenous isotonic saline or sodium bicarbonate solution given before and after the radio-contrast study reduces the risk of CIN [7] (Fig. 15.25).

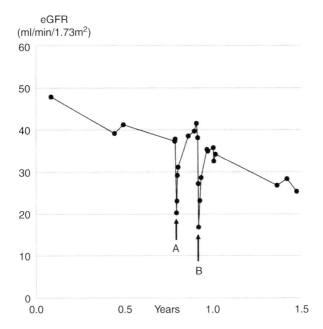

Fig. 15.25 Progressive decline in eGFR in a 60 year-old man with diabetes. At the time labeled *A* he underwent an abdominal CT scan with contrast. An acute drop in eGFR followed. At the time labeled *B* he underwent a coronary angiogram. An identical drop in eGFR occurred. Both episodes of contrast-induced nephropathy had the same severity of injury and time course for recovery. The underlying chronic decline in GFR was not affected in this patient

In magnetic resonance imaging, contrast medium containing the element gadolinium is used. It is para-magnetic and so can affect the tissue behaviour in the magnetic field. Gadolinium is chelated with large organic molecules to avoid the toxicity of gadolinium ions. The complexes are hyperosmolar and excreted by glomerular filtration. If gadolinium-contrast is used in patients with low GFR, the persistently high levels can stimulate a fibrosing reaction in the tissues under the skin and in other organs – nephrogenic systemic fibrosis (NSF). This debilitating and potentially fatal condition is untreatable. Hence a strict GFR limit of >30 ml/min/1.73 m² is applied to the use of contrast containing gadolinium [7].

References

1. Curry NS, Cochran ST, Bissada NK. Cystic renal masses. Am J Roentgenol. 2000;175(2):339–42. http://www.ajronline.org/doi/abs/10.2214/ajr.175.2.1750339.
2. Kermani TA, Crowson CS, Achenbach SJ, Luthra HS. Idiopathic retroperitoneal fibrosis: a retrospective review of clinical presentation, treatment, and outcomes. Mayo Clin Proc. 2011;86(4):297–303. doi:10.4065/mcp.2010.0663. http://www.ncbi.nlm.nih.gov/pmc/articles/PMC3068889/.

3. Smith-Bindman R, Aubin C, Bailitz J, Bengiamin RN, Camargo Jr CA, Corbo J, Dean AJ, Goldstein RB, Griffey RT, Jay GD, Kang TL, Kriesel DR, Ma OJ, Mallin M, Manson W, Melnikow J, Miglioretti DL, Miller SK, Mills LD, Miner JR, Moghadassi M, Noble VE, Press GM, Stoller ML, Valencia VE, Wang J, Wang RC, Cummings SR. Ultrasonography versus computed tomography for suspected nephrolithiasis. N Engl J Med. 2014;371(12):1100–10. doi:10.1056/NEJMoa1404446. http://www.nejm.org/doi/full/10.1056/NEJMoa1404446.
4. Maalouf NM. Approach to the adult kidney stone former. Clin Rev Bone Miner Metab. 2012;10(1):38–49. http://link.springer.com/article/10.1007/s12018-011-9111-9/fulltext.html.
5. Huang JJ, Tseng CC. Emphysematous pyelonephritis: clinicoradiological classification, management, prognosis, and pathogenesis. Arch Intern Med. 2000;160(6):797–805. http://archinte.jamanetwork.com/article.aspx?articleid=485260.
6. Tepel M, Aspelin P, Lameire N. Contrast-induced nephropathy: a clinical and evidence-based approach. Circulation. 2006;113(14):1799–806. doi:10.1161/CIRCULATIONAHA.105.595090. http://circ.ahajournals.org/content/113/14/1799.full.
7. KDIGO Clinical Practice Guideline for Acute Kidney Injury. Contrast-induced AKI. Kidney Int Suppl. 2012;2(1):69–88. doi:10.1038/kisup.2011.34. http://www.ncbi.nlm.nih.gov/pmc/articles/PMC4089629/%5D.

Chapter 16
Should We Do a Kidney Biopsy?

Balancing the Diagnostic Benefits Against the Clinical Risks

Abstract In this chapter we explain:

- Risk assessment when considering a kidney biopsy
- When a kidney biopsy is useful in someone with diabetes

No guidelines or consensus statements have been issued by specialist organisations to help clinicians decide when to perform a kidney biopsy. Therefore the following comments are our personal views, inevitably coloured by our clinical experiences.

'Primum Non Nocere' – First, Do No Harm

Most nephrologists know of patients who have come to serious harm as a result of a kidney biopsy. Even with ultrasound guidance, it is not possible to guide the needle to avoid blood vessels (see Fig. 16.1). Hence, every kidney biopsy causes bleeding; the issue is how much. Published reports state that about 1 in every 100 patients requires a blood transfusion. Unpublished results are likely to be higher. Fatality is much rarer but is a genuine risk that must be considered [1].

Kidney histology is fascinating and beautiful. However, curiosity about what will be found is, on its own, insufficient justification to perform a biopsy. Remember the old saying: 'Curiosity killed the cat'. If you cannot answer the question: "How will the result of this biopsy affect the treatment plan *and* the likely outcome for the patient?" you should reconsider whether to seek the patient's consent.

Although histology may sometimes provide a more precise prognosis, proteinuria and the trend in eGFR are often adequate guides to the patient's future (see Sect. "The clinical significance of haematuria" in page 136). Using the results of the biopsy primarily for academic purposes requires the patient to give explicit consent, as they would for a research study.

Conventional inclusion criteria for considering a biopsy are based upon the likelihood of finding a treatable disease [2]. They include:

- Proteinuria more than 1 g per day (PCR >100 mg/mmol, >1000 mg/g)

© Springer International Publishing Switzerland 2016
H. Rayner et al., *Understanding Kidney Diseases*,
DOI 10.1007/978-3-319-23458-8_16

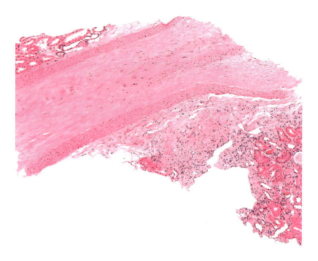

Fig. 16.1 Light micrograph of a section through a renal biopsy specimen showing the wall of a muscular artery. Haematoxylin and eosin ×4

- eGFR declining over weeks or months, with or without haematuria and proteinuria
- Systemic illness with evidence of kidney involvement where a tissue diagnosis is needed

Exclusion criteria are based upon the likelihood of finding irreversible damage. They include:

- Reduced kidney size with thin cortical width
- eGFR declining over years

The risk of bleeding is greater in patients who have:

- high serum urea
- anaemia
- low platelets or abnormal clotting
- anticoagulant or antiplatelet therapy, e.g. clopidogrel

Is It Diabetic Nephropathy?

The 'to biopsy or not to biopsy' dilemma often arises in people with diabetes. As diabetes is so common, it is possible that the patient has an unrelated kidney disease.

First, view the kidneys with an ultrasound scan. Diabetic nephropathy does not affect the ultrasound appearances, other than sometimes by increasing the echogenicity of the cortex so that the differentiation between the cortex and medulla is reduced.

If the ultrasound scan is normal, the following questions are helpful:

1. How long has the patient been diabetic?

   Nephropathy usually only develops once the patient has been diabetic for over 10 years. However, it can sometimes be difficult to estimate exactly how long diabetes has been present as type 2 diabetes can remain asymptomatic for a number of years. The likelihood of nephropathy is greater if there has been a long period of poor glucose control [3].

2. Does the patient have type 1 or type 2 diabetes?

   A renal biopsy is much less likely to reveal pathology other than diabetic nephropathy in someone with type 1 rather than type 2 diabetes.

3. Has there been a change in the rate of decline in GFR?

   A typical rate of decline in GFR in someone with diabetic nephropathy is 3 ml/min/1.73 m^2/year [4]. However, in patients with poorly controlled blood pressure or a long history of poor glucose control the decline can be faster than 10 ml/min/1.73 m^2/year.

   As a rule of thumb, the slower the rate of decline, the less likely the loss will be reversible. A sudden change in the rate of decline is a sign that there has been a change in the underlying disease process which may be treatable.

4. Is there proteinuria or haematuria?

   A patient with reduced GFR due to diabetic nephropathy will usually (but not invariably [5]) have proteinuria with an albumin:creatinine ratio greater than 30 mg/mmol (300 mg/g). Conversely, there is usually no microscopic haematuria, or at most a trace. If there is no protein or both blood and protein on a urine dipstick test, there may be pathology other than diabetic nephropathy.

5. Is the patient hypertensive?

   Diabetic nephropathy typically leads to sodium and water retention and high blood pressure. If the patient has normal blood pressure on no antihypertensive treatment, it may not be diabetic nephropathy.

6. Are there other complications of diabetes?

   The microvascular and macrovascular effects of diabetes are rarely confined to the kidneys. Patients with diabetic nephropathy almost always have retinopathy [3] and often have cardiovascular or peripheral vascular disease.

7. Are there blood tests indicating inflammation?

   Diabetic nephropathy is not an inflammatory disease. If the level of C-reactive protein (CRP) is increased and there is no obvious infection or other cause, the inflammation may be related to a kidney disease. Other immunological tests such as serum immunoglobulins and auto-antibodies can provide further information, although low titres of anti-nuclear and anti-cytoplasmic antibodies may be unrelated to kidney disease.

Patients 16.1 and 16.2 illustrate these points.

Patient 16.1: Crescentic Glomerulonephritis
Mr. Reynolds had had insulin-treated type 2 diabetes for 20 years. Despite good glucose and blood pressure control, his eGFR was progressively declining. He was otherwise well with only background diabetic retinopathy and no cardiovascular disease.

At a routine checkup, his eGFR was found to have dropped much further than expected from the previous trend. The urine dipstick test showed both blood and protein. CRP was 1 mg/L; myeloperoxidase and proteinase 3 ANCA antibodies were not detected.

Stopping the ACE inhibitor treatment did not lead to any improvement. A renal biopsy was performed. The specimen showed a crescentic glomerulonephritis (see Figs. 14.6 and 14.7).

He responded well to treatment with cyclophosphamide and prednisolone and his eGFR increased to near its previous level (Fig. 16.2).

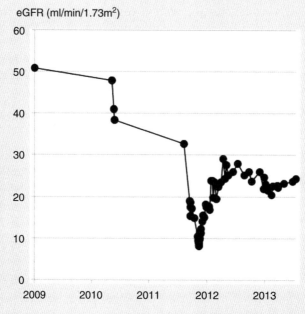

Fig. 16.2 Fall in eGFR due to crescentic glomerulonephritis and rise following treatment

Patient 16.2: Interstitial Nephritis

Mrs. Clarkson had type 2 diabetes, well controlled with metformin. She was troubled by gastro-oesophageal reflux and started taking a proton-pump inhibitor (PPI, omeprazole) for her symptoms. Six months later, her GFR started to decline rapidly. Her urine contained no blood or protein. Her kidneys looked normal on an ultrasound scan. Full blood count (including eosinophils), CRP and immunological tests were normal.

A renal biopsy showed acute interstitial nephritis, most likely caused by the PPI (Fig. 16.3).

The PPI was replaced by an H_2-receptor antagonist (ranitidine) and she was treated with 30 mg prednisolone per day.

Her GFR steadily improved, although her glucose control became so erratic on the corticosteroids that she required insulin temporarily. She was left with some residual loss of kidney function (Fig. 16.4).

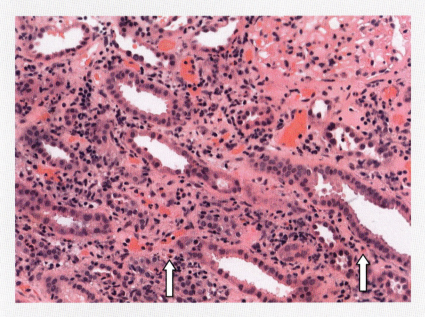

Fig. 16.3 Kidney biopsy section showing typical appearances of interstitial nephritis. There is an infiltration of inflammatory cells between the tubules, mainly lymphocytes with some eosinophils (*arrows*). The glomerulus (*top right*) is normal. Haematoxylin and eosin ×200

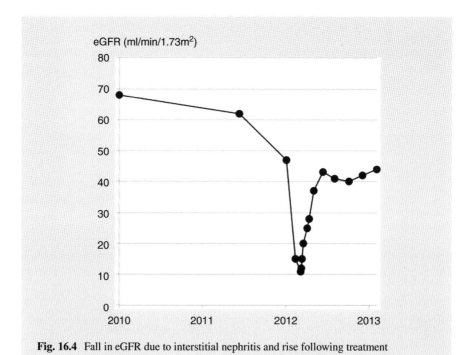

Fig. 16.4 Fall in eGFR due to interstitial nephritis and rise following treatment

References

1. Corapi KM, Chen JL, Balk EM, Gordon CE. Bleeding complications of native kidney biopsy: a systematic review and meta-analysis. Am J Kidney Dis. 2012;60(1):62–73. doi:10.1053/j.ajkd.2012.02.330. Epub 2012 Apr 24. http://www.ajkd.org/article/S0272-6386(12)00558-6/abstract.
2. Dhaun N, Bellamy CO, Cattran DC, Kluth DC. Utility of renal biopsy in the clinical management of renal disease. Kidney Int. 2014;85(5):1039–48. doi:10.1038/ki.2013.512. Epub 2014 Jan 8. http://www.nature.com/ki/journal/v85/n5/full/ki2013512a.html.
3. Pallayova M, Mohammed A, Langman G, Taheri S, Dasgupta I. Predicting non-diabetic renal disease in type 2 diabetic adults: the value of glycated hemoglobin. J Diabetes Complications. 2015;29(5):718–23. doi:10.1016/j.jdiacomp.2014.12.005. pii: S1056-8727(14)00401-2. http://www.ncbi.nlm.nih.gov/pubmed/25633572.
4. Ruggenenti P, Porrini EL, Gaspari F, Motterlini N, Cannata A, Carrara F, Cella C, Ferrari S, Stucchi N, Parvanova A, Iliev I, Dodesini AR, Trevisan R, Bossi A, Zaletel J, Remuzzi G, GFR Study Investigators. Glomerular hyperfiltration and renal disease progression in type 2 diabetes. Diabetes Care. 2012;35(10):2061–8. Epub 2012 Jul 6. http://care.diabetesjournals.org/content/35/10/2061.long.
5. Perkins BA, Ficociello LH, Roshan B, Warram JH, Krolewski AS. In patients with type 1 diabetes and new-onset microalbuminuria the development of advanced chronic kidney disease may not require progression to proteinuria. Kidney Int. 2010;77(1):57–64. doi:10.1038/ki.2009.399. http://www.nature.com/ki/journal/v77/n1/full/ki2009399a.html.

Chapter 17
Make a Plan

When and How to Prepare for End-Stage Kidney Disease

Abstract In this chapter we explain:

- Risk assessment using eGFR and proteinuria
- Competing risks of dialysis and death
- How a patient's future may be predicted by their eGFR graph
- How patients are prepared for end-stage kidney failure
- Treatment options for someone with end-stage kidney failure
- When dialysis should be started

Once you have made a diagnosis of kidney disease, the next step is to agree a treatment plan with the patient. We do not provide guidelines for the management of individual conditions in this book. However, there are some principles that apply generally to the planning of treatment for kidney disease.

Understanding Risk and Predicting the Future

eGFR and proteinuria are useful for assessing a patient's prognosis. Patients with a low eGFR and proteinuria have an increased risk of end-stage kidney disease and of death, largely due to cardiovascular disease.

Figure 17.1 shows the relative risk of death for people in four age categories according to their eGFR and albuminuria. In each chart, the columns show someone's risk of death compared to someone in the same age category with normal kidney function and no albuminuria. The reference category is eGFR = 75–89 ml/min/1.73 m^2 with urine dipstick showing no proteinuria or an albumin:creatinine ratio <1.1 mg/mmol (<10 mg/g).

One can draw a number of conclusions from these charts. Firstly, the lower someone's eGFR and the greater their amount of albuminuria, the greater is their risk of death. eGFR and albuminuria each increases the risk in its own right. This applies to all age categories, implying that reduced eGFR and albuminuria are not inevitable features of ageing but represent markers of disease.

Secondly, the increase in relative risk is large, especially in the youngest age category. Someone aged 18–54 years with an eGFR of 15–29 and no albuminuria is

© Springer International Publishing Switzerland 2016
H. Rayner et al., *Understanding Kidney Diseases*,
DOI 10.1007/978-3-319-23458-8_17

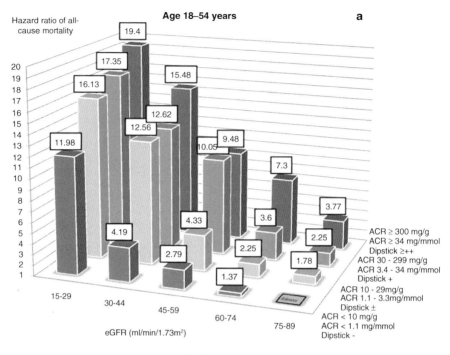

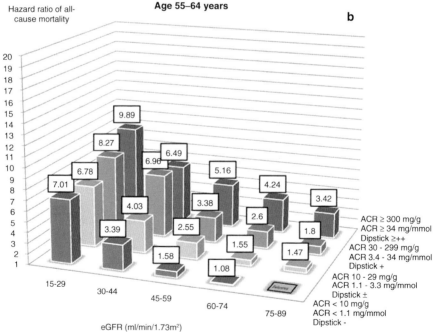

Fig. 17.1 Risk of mortality associated with eGFR and albuminuria by age category (**a** = 18–54 years, **b** = 55–64 years, **c** = 65–74 years, **d** = 75+ years) (Drawn using data from Hallan et al. [1])

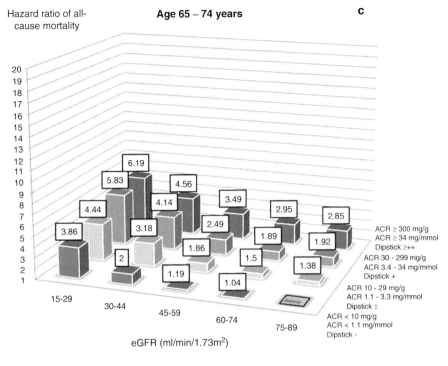

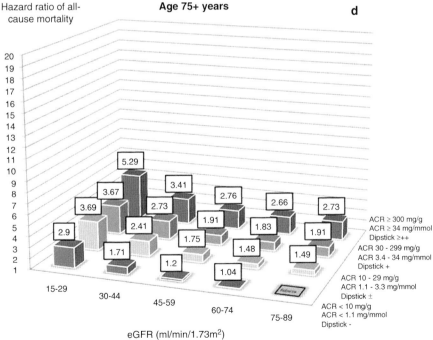

Fig. 17.1 (continued)

12 times more likely to die over the next 5.8 years than someone with an eGFR 75–89. Similarly, someone with a urine albumin:creatinine ratio >34 mg/mmol (ACR >300 mg/g, dipstick ++ or more) but normal eGFR is nearly four times more likely to die. Combining the two factors increases the risk nearly 20 times.

Thirdly, the relative risk of death associated with reduced eGFR and albuminuria gets smaller with age. However, as the underlying risk of death in the reference group increases with age, the effect of reduced eGFR and albuminuria on the number of people dying per year is greater in the older age groups.

What are the implications of these findings for clinical practice? It is important to remember that these are measurements of the risk of death *associated with* reduced eGFR and albuminuria. That does not mean that reduced kidney function or albuminuria in some way *cause* the deaths, or that increasing eGFR or reducing albuminuria will necessarily reduce the risk of death.

The effect of reduced eGFR on outcomes has been studied in kidney donors. When one of their kidneys is removed, the donors go from normal to CKD stage 2 or 3. Does this reduced eGFR increase their risk of future cardiovascular disease? The answer seems to be 'no'. Comparing Canadian kidney donors with the healthiest segment of the general population there is no increase in the risk of major cardiovascular events over the next 10 years [2]. However, kidney donors do have twice the risk of developing high blood pressure or pre-eclampsia in pregnancy (11 % versus 5 %) [3].

Studies in animal models of more advanced CKD suggest a causal link between reduced kidney function and heart disease such as left ventricular hypertrophy. Kidney tubular epithelium is the main producer of a protein called Klotho that has anti-aging properties. It is released into the circulation like a hormone and its levels decline in CKD. One of its actions is to bind the uraemic toxin indoxyl sulfate which is cardiotoxic. In CKD, levels of Klotho are reduced and so too is its cardioprotective effect [4].

Knowing about your risk of dying is only useful if something can be done about it. The opportunity to alter the natural history of disease is more limited as people get older. Nonetheless, treatment to a target systolic blood pressure of 150/80 mmHg in people aged over 80 years who are otherwise well reduces the rate of death, stroke and heart failure within 1–2 years [5]. On the other hand, over-aggressive treatment of blood pressure in elderly people with other comorbidities increases the risk of falls and harm.

Finally, the wishes of the patient must be taken into account when deciding how much attention to give to these risk factors. An elderly person suffering from a number of long-term conditions may give a much higher priority to improving the quality of their life than its length.

Competing Risks: Dialysis or Death?

The risk of developing end-stage kidney disease can be gauged from three factors: age, eGFR and the level of proteinuria. Although the type of disease causing the kidney failure does play a part, when considering people with the same pathological condition the prognosis is largely determined by these three factors.

Studies of populations of patients with CKD show that, for a given level of eGFR, the risk of dying before reaching the need to start dialysis increases steadily with age (Fig. 17.2).

Fig. 17.2 Competing risks of end-stage kidney disease (ESRD) and death according to age and eGFR for people with chronic kidney disease (Based upon Refs. [6, 7])

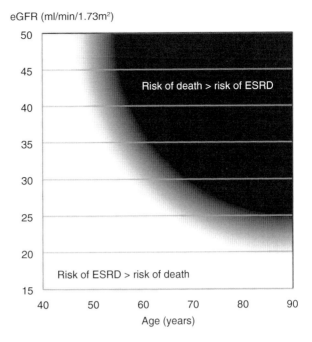

Damage to the glomerular endothelial cells reflects damage to the endothelium of microvessels elsewhere in the body. This includes the vasa vasorum that provide the blood supply to the walls of large arteries. This may explain the link between albuminuria, uraemia and cardiovascular disease [8]. Measuring albuminuria or proteinuria is a useful way of measuring the health of someone's blood vessels and with it their risk of renal failure and death.

Data from a community mass-screening programme in Japan showed how the risk of renal failure increased with the level of proteinuria [9]. Even small amounts were significant; having + proteinuria on dipstick testing increased the risk of end-stage renal failure by 1.9 times in men and 2.4 times in women.

For older patients, a validated risk score that incorporates nine clinical variables gives an assessment of the risk of death within 5 years before reaching end-stage kidney disease [10].

Risk analyses such as these are very helpful for identifying categories of people who may benefit from more intensive treatment. They are less useful for planning the treatment for individual patients. Unlike in most chronic medical conditions where we can offer only probabilities of what might happen in the future, with kidney disease we can often make a prediction for the individual patient.

Prognostication: "Be Prepared"

Many patients attend the kidney clinic anxious they may need to start dialysis. The eGFR graph can be very helpful for judging if that is true and, if so, when it is likely to happen (Patient 17.1).

Patient 17.1: Projection of the eGFR Graph to Predict the Need for Dialysis

Mr. Arnold had been followed regularly in the clinic for his CKD. Over a 9-year period his eGFR had declined by 15 ml/min/1.73 m² (Fig. 17.3).

To predict the future, a trendline was projected on the chart (Fig. 17.4).

If Mr. Arnold's loss of kidney function continued at the same rate, he would reach an eGFR of 10 ml/min/1.73 m² at the age of 97 years. He was very relieved to know that he did not need to worry about having dialysis for the foreseeable future.

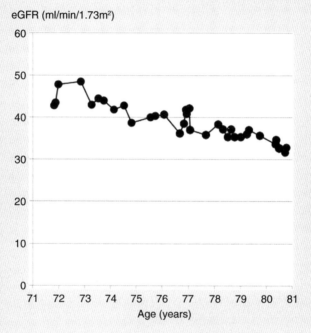

Fig. 17.3 Decline in eGFR by approximately 1.5 ml/min/1.73 m²/year

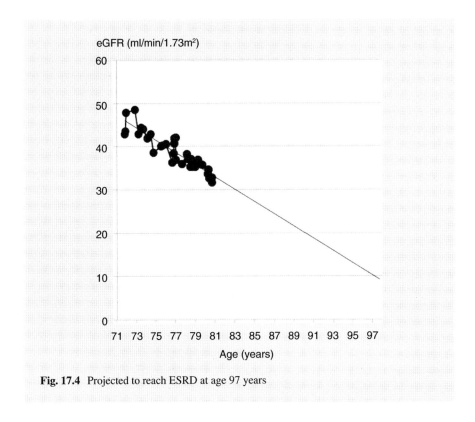

Fig. 17.4 Projected to reach ESRD at age 97 years

When the trendline on the eGFR graph indicates that someone is likely to need dialysis, care should be planned accordingly. We can learn how to do this from the example of another condition in which health needs are predictable – pregnancy.

Ante-natal classes are provided to help parents prepare for an event that will transform their lives. Like having your first baby, renal failure and dialysis can disrupt your sleep and leave you feeling exhausted. Like bringing up a child, dialysis limits your freedom and continues week-in, week-out for years.

Education and care of patients with advanced kidney failure is provided by a team of professionals, coordinated around the needs of the patient. They address issues that also feature in ante-natal classes, such as:

- Choice of medical treatment
- Symptom control and self-care
- Psychological support
- Involvement of carers and relatives

The decision about when to transfer care to this multidisciplinary team is determined by the time needed to prepare for dialysis or a kidney transplant. In pregnancy there are 9 months to prepare; in kidney failure a year is ideal, possibly longer if a transplant is the preferred option. Asking the 'surprise' question is helpful: "Would you be surprised if this patient needed to start dialysis within the next year?"

Fig. 17.5 Examples of differences in the rate of decline of GFR between three patients. Transfer to the multiprofessional team occurred at different levels of eGFR to allow at least a year for preparation for transplantation or dialysis

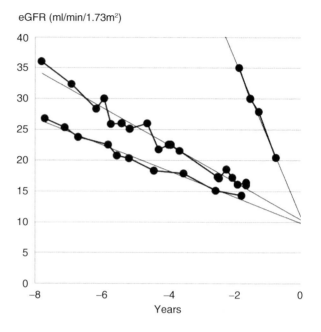

The eGFR graph helps answer this question. The rate of decline in eGFR varies between patients so there is no single value of eGFR when planning should start. Instead, projecting the eGFR graph forwards to 10 ml/min/1.73 m² will give an estimate of the time remaining (Fig. 17.5).

It is wise to have a lower limit of 15 ml/min/1.73 m² for referral. When the remaining kidney function is this low, an unpredictable acute illness can easily precipitate the need for dialysis. When a transplant is planned as the first renal replacement treatment, it is usually carried out when eGFR falls below 15 ml/min/1.73 m² to avoid the risk of unplanned dialysis.

The following story (Patient 17.2) illustrates the kinds of problems that may be addressed during the period of preparation.

Patient 17.2: Planning Dialysis

Mr. Fielding was a 72-year-old retired businessman who divided his time between the family home in Birmingham and a business in Wales. His type 2 diabetes was well treated with insulin but his blood pressure was not well controlled. He reported home systolic blood pressure readings between 165 and 170 mmHg despite taking four antihypertensive drugs.

His kidney function had steadily deteriorated through the late 1990s due to diabetic nephropathy. At a clinic visit in February 2003 his eGFR graph predicted that he would reach end-stage kidney failure in 2005 (Fig. 17.6).

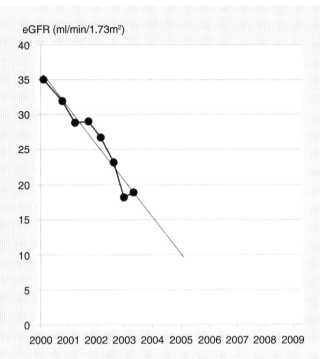

Fig. 17.6 Projected decline in eGFR using trendline

We talked at length about what type of dialysis he would wish to have, a kidney transplant being inappropriate because of angina. In the end he settled on peritoneal dialysis, which would suit his need to return to Wales at regular intervals to manage the business. As he had had no previous abdominal surgery, the peritoneal dialysis catheter could be inserted under a local anaesthetic nearer the time.

A year later, the graph showed that his eGFR had declined as predicted (Fig. 17.7).

His care was transferred to the multi-disciplinary predialysis clinic where he could see the specialist nurses, dietitian, anaemia nurse, social worker and consultant at the same visit.

Because of his reduced GFR, his insulin requirements had declined and he was having hypoglycaemia at night. His insulin dose was reduced accordingly. Otherwise, he was asymptomatic and we agreed not to make further preparations for dialysis for the time being. However, he decided that the time had come for him to sell up the business in Wales.

By 2006, he had become more breathless due to anaemia and was treated with erythropoietin. Then, tragically, his wife became very ill. Having sold the business, Mr Fielding was able to devote himself to caring for his wife. She sadly died in late 2006.

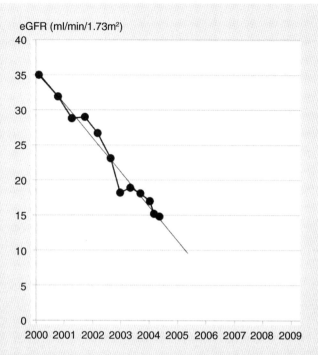

Fig. 17.7 Continued decline in eGFR along the projected trendline

During this time, his eGFR had been stable, confounding our predictions that he would need dialysis (Fig. 17.8). He was not critical of us; indeed he was grateful that we had helped him make the decision to sell his business in Wales as this had enabled him to care for his wife throughout her illness.

After the death of his wife, Mr. Fielding's physical and emotional health declined. His eyesight deteriorated and he moved into sheltered accommodation. It became clear that haemodialysis would be more suitable for him than peritoneal dialysis. An arteriovenous fistula was formed in his left forearm in September 2008. An operation in March 2009 improved the blood flow so that the fistula could be cannulated when the time came to start dialysis.

In 2009, 4 years later than predicted, he became more symptomatic of kidney failure. His eGFR reached 7.1, urea 44.9 mmol/L (126 mg/dL), calcium 2.17 mmol/L (8.7 mg/dL), phosphate 2.82 mmol/L (8.7 mg/dL), venous bicarbonate 15.1 mmol/L (mEq/L) (Fig. 17.9). Dialysis was started as a routine outpatient procedure using his arteriovenous fistula.

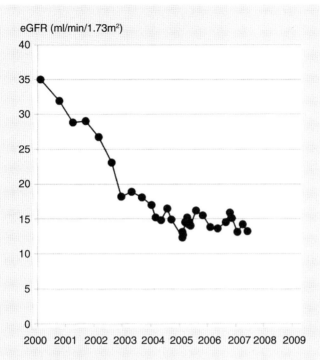

Fig. 17.8 Slowing of decline in eGFR

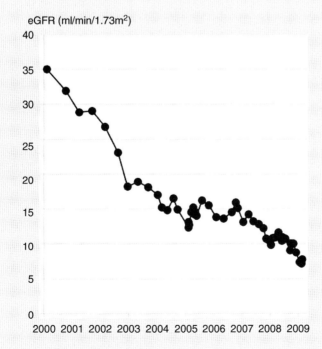

Fig. 17.9 eGFR decline to the start of dialysis

Writing Letters to Patients

Guidance from the governing body for doctors in the UK, the General Medical Council, states that doctors should:

- Give patients the information they want or need in a way they can understand
- Support patients in caring for themselves to improve and maintain their health

The eGFR graph is the best way of giving patients information about their kidney function in a way they can understand. A copy of the graph should be given to the patient, either during the consultation or enclosed with the clinic letter.

The letter written following the consultation is a great opportunity to support patients in caring for their health. This is best achieved by writing the letter directly to the patient. A copy of this letter is sent to the General Practitioner so that the information and advice can be reiterated by the Primary Care team.

Some tips for writing good letters to patients:

- Use simpler words without losing the meaning, e.g., 'kidney' rather than 'renal'
- Do not use medical terminology in the body of the text unless you are certain that the patient will understand it. Words may be misinterpreted, e.g., 'chronic' may be interpreted as meaning 'severe'
- Avoid acronyms such as AKI, CKD and ESRD
- Separate medical terms into a diagnosis or problem list. This allows patients to conduct further research into their condition if they wish
- Include a medication list using English rather than Latin (e.g., bd) and highlight any changes, e.g., 'furosemide **increased** to 80 mg twice a day'
- Use graphs wherever you can to describe changes in results, e.g., eGFR, albumin

Do not dictate the letter in the same way that you would talk to the patient:

- Remove words and phrases that add little meaning, e.g., 'actually', 'really'
- Use shorter sentences – e.g., fewer if's, and's & but's
- Have one topic per paragraph

Writing good letters to patients is not easy; it improves with practice and from patient feedback. However, once you are confident writing them, you will never want to go back to your old ways, and your patients will benefit greatly.

Choosing Treatment: Transplant, Haemodialysis, Peritoneal Dialysis or No Dialysis?

For most patients with end-stage kidney disease it is an easy decision to have renal replacement therapy (RRT). Best of all is to arrange for a transplant from a living donor before dialysis is needed – a pre-emptive transplant. This can be a kidney alone or, for some patients with diabetes, a kidney and a pancreas.

If dialysis is felt to be the right choice, is there any difference between haemodialysis or peritoneal dialysis? Studies have not shown a consistent survival advantage for either type of dialysis. PD offers greater independence from the dialysis unit but imposes a greater responsibility on the patient. The eventual decision should be determined mainly by the patient's choice. Some patients find written or web-based information helpful, such as at http://www.nhs.uk/conditions/Dialysis/Pages/Introduction.aspx.

For some patients the decision whether to have dialysis is more difficult. The benefits of the treatment may be outweighed by its burdens. The journey back and forth to the dialysis unit three times every week can be exhausting. Patients may feel unwell during the treatment and tired for hours afterwards [11]. Patient with severe cognitive impairment may be made more confused by dialysis. Patients who are older, frail and have co-morbidities may opt to have their symptoms controlled with conservative care rather than to start or continue with dialysis [12].

When Should Dialysis Be Started?

Dialysis should be started when the benefits outweigh the harm and inconvenience. The 'Initiating Dialysis Early And Late' (IDEAL) study reassures us that starting dialysis earlier than this is not beneficial [13]. In the trial, the start of dialysis was delayed by an average of 6 months in the later start group, eGFR falling to 7.2 ml/min/1.73 m^2 compared to 9.0 in the early start group.

In the UK, the mean eGFR at the start of dialysis is 8.5 ml/min/1.73 m^2. This is much lower than in the US, a difference only partly explained by differences between UK and US patients.

Oedema, both pulmonary and peripheral, which cannot be controlled with high doses or a combination of diuretics, is a common reason to start dialysis. Increasing tiredness, loss of appetite and finally nausea may prompt the start.

A rise in serum phosphate and fall in serum bicarbonate, in addition to a high urea and low estimated GFR, are useful signs that the true GFR is low enough to warrant dialysis (Patient 17.3).

Patient 17.3: Starting Dialysis by Symptoms Rather Than Numbers
Mr. Shaw was a retired man aged 70 years. He felt well and was able to do all his usual activities. He had a good appetite and ate well. He took regular exercise and had not lost any body weight or muscle bulk.

He was taking sodium bicarbonate 1 g twice daily, alfacalcidol 0.25 mcg daily, erythropoietin and no dietary phosphate binders. He had chosen to have haemodialysis and had a functioning arterio-venous fistula in his left forearm.

He was seen monthly in clinic. His eGFR had declined from 7.5 to 5.0 ml/min/1.73 m² over last 12 months. Table 17.1 shows his blood results.

Table 17.1 Laboratory results from Mr. Shaw

		Normal range	Non-SI units
Sodium	145 mmol/L	133–146	145 mEq/L
Potassium	5.2 mmol/L	3.5–5.3	5.2 mEq/L
Urea	34.7 mmol/L	2.5–7.8	BUN 97 mg/dL
Creatinine	850 mcmol/L	64–111	9.6 mg/dL
eGFR	5.0 ml/min/1.73 m²		
Bicarbonate	22.5 mmol/L	22.0–29.0	22.5 mEq/L
Albumin	39 g/L	35–50	3.9 g/dL
Calcium (corrected for serum albumin)	2.51 mmol/L	2.20–2.60	10.0 mEq/L
Phosphate	1.40 mmol/L	0.80–1.50	4.3 mEq/L
Haemoglobin	111 g/L	135–180	11.1 g/dL

Despite the low eGFR, dialysis was not started. The true GFR was likely higher than the estimated GFR because of his good muscle bulk. The relatively high urea (BUN) was related to his good protein intake

Care of the Whole Person

It would be wrong not to emphasise the importance of psychosocial factors in the progression and treatment of kidney failure.

Observational studies have shown a strong association between the amount of social support a person has and their risk of developing kidney failure [14] and of having a poorer quality of life and dying when on dialysis [15].

Anxiety and depression are common amongst people with kidney disease. Being depressed is one of the strongest markers for mortality in people on dialysis [16].

Replacing kidney function is only one part of the care needed by people with kidney failure. Support in the form of exercise programs [17] and psychological therapies [18] should form an important part of the package of care (Fig. 17.10).

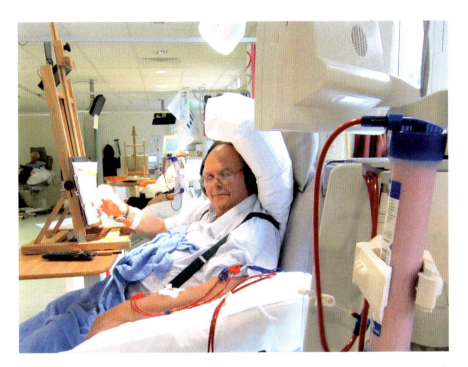

Fig. 17.10 Dialysis is one part of holistic treatment for kidney failure. Time spent having dialysis can be put to good use with activities such as exercise or, as in this unit, art lessons. The British Kidney Patient Association, a charity that supports people with kidney disease, funded this project

References

1. Hallan SI, Matsushita K, Sang Y, Mahmoodi BK, Black C, Ishani A, Kleefstra N, Naimark D, Roderick P, Tonelli M, Wetzels JFM, Astor BC, Gansevoort RT, Levin A, Wen C-P, Coresh J, for the CKD Prognosis Consortium. Age and the association of kidney measures with mortality and end-stage renal disease. JAMA. 2012;308(22):2349–60. doi:10.1001/jama.2012.16817. http://jama.jamanetwork.com/article.aspx?articleid=1387683.
2. Garg AX, Meirambayeva A, Huang A, Kim J, Prasad GVR, Knoll G, et al. Cardiovascular disease in kidney donors: matched cohort study. BMJ. 2012;344, e1203. http://www.bmj.com/content/344/bmj.e1203.
3. Garg AX, Nevis IF, McArthur E, Sontrop JM, Koval JJ, Lam NN, Hildebrand AM, Reese PP, Storsley L, Gill JS, Segev DL, Habbous S, Bugeja A, Knoll GA, Dipchand C, Monroy-Cuadros M, Lentine KL, for the DONOR Network. Gestational hypertension and preeclampsia in living kidney donors. N Engl J Med. 2014. doi:10.1056/NEJMoa1408932. http://www.nejm.org/doi/full/10.1056/NEJMoa1408932

4. Fu H, Liu Y. Loss of Klotho in CKD breaks one's heart. J Am Soc Nephrol 2015;26(10): 2305-7. doi:10.1681/ASN.2015020200. http://jasn.asnjournals.org/content/early/2015/03/23/ASN.2015020200

5. Beckett NS, Peters R, Fletcher AE, Staessen JA, Liu L, Dumitrascu D, Stoyanovsky V, Antikainen RL, Nikitin Y, Anderson C, Belhani A, Forette F, Rajkumar C, Thijs L, Banya W, Bulpitt CJ, HYVET Study Group. Treatment of hypertension in patients 80 years of age or older. N Engl J Med. 2008;358:1887–98. http://www.nejm.org/doi/full/10.1056/NEJMoa0801369#t=article.

6. De Nicola L, Minutolo R, Chiodini P, Borrelli S, Zoccali C, Postorino M, Iodice C, Nappi F, Fuiano G, Gallo C, Conte G, the Italian Society of Nephrology Study Group 'TArget Blood pressure LEvels (TABLE) in CKD. The effect of increasing age on the prognosis of non-dialysis patients with chronic kidney disease receiving stable nephrology care. Kidney Int. 2012;82:482–8. doi:10.1038/ki.2012.174. http://www.nature.com/ki/journal/v82/n4/full/ki2012174a.html.

7. O'Hare AM, Choi AI, Bertenthal D, Bacchetti P, Garg AX, Kaufman JS, Walter LC, Mehta KM, Steinman MA, Allon M, McClellan WM, Landefeld CS. Age affects outcomes in chronic kidney disease. J Am Soc Nephrol. 2007;18:2758–65. doi:10.1681/ASN.2007040422. http://jasn.asnjournals.org/content/18/10/2758.long.

8. Harper SJ, Bates DO. Endothelial permeability in uremia. Kidney Int. 2003;63:S41–4. doi:10.1046/j.1523-1755.63.s84.15.x. http://www.nature.com/ki/journal/v63/n84s/abs/4493766a.html.

9. Iseki K, Ikemiya Y, Iseki C, Takishita S. Proteinuria and the risk of developing end-stage renal disease. Kidney Int. 2003;63:1468–74. http://www.nature.com/ki/journal/v63/n4/full/4493578a.html.

10. Bansal N, Katz R, De Boer IH, Peralta CA, Fried LF, Siscovick DS, Rifkin DE, Hirsch C, Cummings SR, Harris TB, Kritchevsky SB, Sarnak MJ, Shlipak MG, Joachim H. Development and validation of a model to predict 5-year risk of death without ESRD among older adults with CKD. Clin J Am Soc Nephrol. 2015;10(3):363–71. doi:10.2215/CJN.04650514. http://cjasn.asnjournals.org/content/early/2015/02/18/CJN.04650514.abstract.

11. Rayner HC, Zepel L, Fuller DS, Morgenstern H, Karaboyas A, Culleton BF, Mapes DL, Lopes AA, Gillespie BW, Hasegawa T, Saran R, Tentori F, Hecking M, Pisoni RL, Robinson BM. Recovery time, quality of life, and mortality in hemodialysis patients: the Dialysis Outcomes and Practice Patterns Study (DOPPS). Am J Kidney Dis. 2014;64(1):86–94. doi:10.1053/j.ajkd.2014.01.014. Epub 2014 Feb 14. http://www.ajkd.org/article/S0272-6386(14)00031-6/abstract.

12. Okamoto I, Tonkin-Crine S, Rayner H, Murtagh FEM, Farrington K, Caskey F, Tomson C, Loud F, Greenwood R, O'Donoghue DJ, Roderick P. Conservative care for ESRD in the United Kingdom: a national survey. Clin J Am Soc Nephrol. 2015;10(1):120–6. doi:10.2215/CJN.05000514. http://cjasn.asnjournals.org/content/early/2014/11/10/CJN.05000514.abstract.

13. Cooper BA, Branley P, Bulfone L, Collins JF, Craig JC, Fraenkel MB, Harris A, Johnson DW, Kesselhut J, Li JJ, Luxton G, Pilmore A, Tiller DJ, Harris DC, Pollock CA, for the IDEAL Study. A randomized, controlled trial of early versus late initiation of dialysis. N Engl J Med. 2010;363:609–19. doi:10.1056/NEJMoa1000552. http://www.nejm.org/doi/full/10.1056/NEJMoa1000552.

14. Dunkler D, Kohl M, Heinze G, Teo KK, Rosengren A, Pogue J, Gao P, Gerstein H, Yusuf S, Oberbauer R, Mann JF. Modifiable lifestyle and social factors affect chronic kidney disease in high-risk individuals with type 2 diabetes mellitus. Kidney Int. 2015;87(4):784–91. doi:10.1038/ki.2014.370. Epub 2014 Dec 10. http://www.nature.com/ki/journal/v87/n4/full/ki2014370a.html.

15. Untas A, Thumma J, Rascle N, Rayner H, Mapes D, Lopes AA, Fukuhara S, Akizawa T, Morgenstern H, Robinson BM, Pisoni RL, Combe C. The associations of social support and other psychosocial factors with mortality and quality of life in the dialysis outcomes and practice patterns study. Clin J Am Soc Nephrol. 2011;6(1):142–52. doi:10.2215/CJN.02340310. http://www.ncbi.nlm.nih.gov/pmc/articles/PMC3022236http://www.ncbi.nlm.nih.gov/pmc/articles/PMC3022236.

16. Lopes AA, Bragg J, Young E, Goodkin D, Mapes D, Combe C, Piera L, Held P, Gillespie B, Port FK. Depression as a predictor of mortality and hospitalization among hemodialysis patients in the United States and Europe. Kidney Int. 2002;62(1):199–207. http://www.nature.com/ki/journal/v62/n1/full/4493090a.html.
17. Jung T-D, Park S-H. Intradialytic exercise programs for hemodialysis patients. Chonnam Med J. 2011;47(2):61–5. doi:10.4068/cmj.2011.47.2.61. http://www.ncbi.nlm.nih.gov/pmc/articles/PMC3214879/.
18. Cukor D, Ver Halen N, Asher DR, Coplan JD, Weedon J, Wyka KE, Saggi SJ, Kimmel PL. Psychosocial intervention improves depression, quality of life, and fluid adherence in hemodialysis. J Am Soc Nephrol. 2014;25:196–206. doi:10.1681/ASN.2012111134. http://jasn.asnjournals.org/content/25/1/196.abstract.

Chapter 18
Renal Replacement Therapy

Common Problems in Dialysis and Transplant Patients

Abstract In this chapter we explain:

- How to assess an arteriovenous fistula
- Peritoneal dialysis catheter problems
- Fluid overload and volume assessment in a dialysis patient
- Causes of a decline in kidney transplant function
- How infections change with time after transplantation
- Malignant disease related to immunosuppression

There are three types of renal replacement therapy – haemodialysis, peritoneal dialysis and a kidney transplant. In this chapter, we explain some clinical aspects of these treatments that may be encountered by a non-specialist doctor, either incidentally when seeing the patient for another problem or in the emergency department.

Haemodialysis

Haemodialysis involves removing blood from the body and passing it though an artificial kidney. This 'dialyser' contains thousands of semi-permeable hollow fibres. Blood flows through the fibres and back to the patient while dialysis fluid flows around the fibres in the opposite direction. Diffusion and ultrafiltration occur across the fibre membrane to remove waste products and excess fluid and correct electrolyte abnormalities. Adequate dialysis is typically achieved by having three treatments per week, each four hours long every week.

Vascular Access

Vascular access, which enables blood to be passed through the dialyser, is a crucial issue in haemodialysis. The ideal method is to insert a large needle into an arteriovenous (AV) fistula or graft. Second best is to insert a catheter into a large vein.

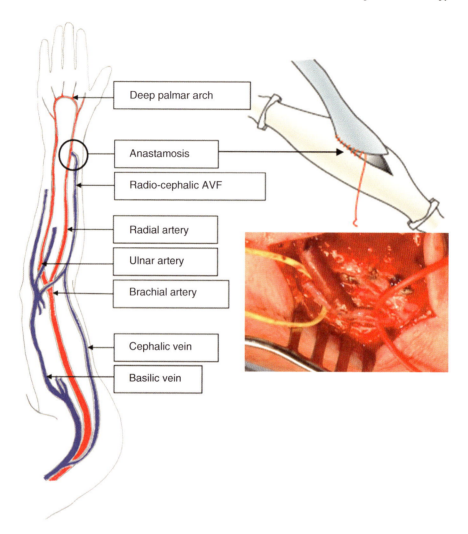

Fig. 18.1 The anatomy of an arteriovenous fistula (AVF). The ideal site for the anastomosis is between the radial artery and the cephalic vein near the wrist, as shown here. Blood returns up the vein rather than continuing into the hand. Perfusion of the hand is normally maintained by flow in the deep palmar arch via a branch from the ulnar artery. Other options for an anastomosis are between the brachial artery and the cephalic vein and between the brachial artery and the basilic vein

An AV fistula is created by joining an artery to an adjacent vein (Fig. 18.1). Strictly speaking, the fistula is the anastomosis but the word is used to refer to the enlarged vein. If an anastomosis is not feasible, a piece of artificial vessel – a graft – may be inserted between the artery and vein.

The increased pressure in the vein causes it to enlarge and develop thickened walls. Over time and with repeated needling, the fistula vein can become massively enlarged.

Fig. 18.2 Ischaemia of the thumb, index and middle fingers caused by the 'stealing' of blood from the radial side of the hand by a radio-cephalic arteriovenous fistula. Flow from the ulnar artery into the deep palmar arch was restricted by atherosclerotic disease. The red wristband warns against venepuncture and blood pressure measurement in the fistula arm

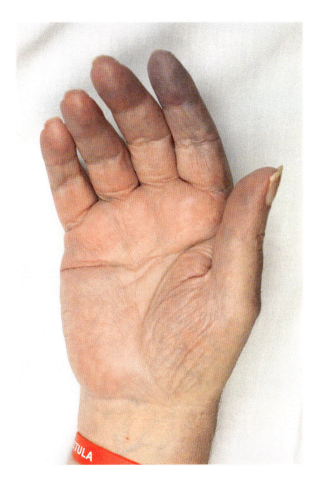

The main problems that arise with an AV fistula are [1]:

- Infection – cellulitis or superficial pustules
- Steal syndrome – reduced perfusion of the distal part of a limb when collateral flow to the extremity cannot compensate for blood diverted to the fistula (Fig. 18.2)
- Ischaemic painful polyneuropathy – commoner with an upper arm fistula and in patients with diabetes or vascular disease
- High output cardiac failure – uncommon but may require the fistula to be tied off
- Clotting – usually due to slow flow caused by a stenosis in the fistula vein; requires urgent specialist attention to increase the chances that the fistula can be salvaged
- Stenosis and aneurysm – often occur together, the aneurysm forming upstream of a stenosis. A rapidly growing aneurysm covered with thin or dusky skin may rupture and requires urgent specialist attention

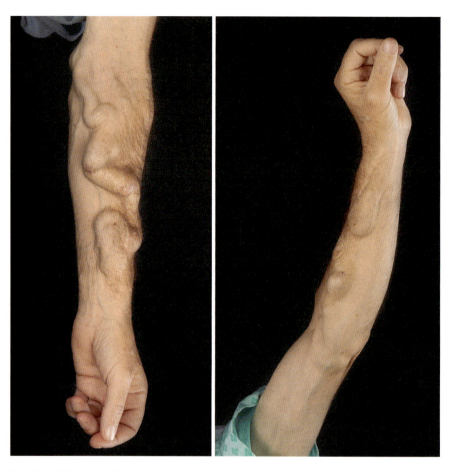

Fig. 18.3 This large radiocephalic fistula is shown with the arm dependent (*left*) and then elevated (*right*). On elevation, the fistula collapses completely except for two distended sections where the vessel wall has been weakened by repeated needling. These were soft, indicating that there was no stenosis obstructing flow. The dilated section near the scar caused by the anastamosis operation showed an arterial pulse wave transmitted from the radial artery. For a video of this examination go to vimeo.com/123945414

Clinical evaluation of a fistula can identify the site of a stenosis. The commonest site is near the anastamosis because the surgical wound stimulates fibrosis in the vein. The stenosis reduces the flow into the fistula, weakening the thrill that can be felt and the bruit that can be heard.

Stenosis in the vein downstream of the fistula increases the pressure in the fistula. Normal fistula pressure is about 35 mmHg; if there is a stenosis, the pressure may be over 100 mmHg. This can be detected by elevating the arm. When the arm is above the head, blood should drain into the right atrium with little resistance to flow and the fistula should collapse. If there is a central stenosis, the fistula vein does not collapse and feels hard and pulsatile (Fig. 18.3).

During dialysis, blood is pumped through the artificial kidney at speeds of about 300 ml/min. If there is a stenosis in the vein downstream of the fistula, blood pumped back into the fistula cannot all escape up the arm. Instead some recirculates round and round the dialysis circuit (Patient 18.1). The patient appears to be dialysing normally but potassium, urea and other toxins are not cleared [2]. The patient may present later as an emergency with a dangerously high serum potassium concentration. Urgent radiological imaging and intervention are needed to dilate the vein, prevent the fistula clotting and restore effective clearance on dialysis.

Patient 18.1: Recirculation Due to Arteriovenous Fistula Stenosis
The dialysis nurses were increasingly concerned about Mr. Trellis' fistula. The blood flow rate during dialysis was normal but the post-dialysis urea and potassium concentrations were 28 and 5.2 mmol/L (BUN=78 mg/dL, K^+=5.2 mEq/L) compared to the usual 15 and 3.5 (42 mg/dL, 3.5 mEq/L) respectively. The monitor of recirculation built into the dialysis machine suggested that the percentage of blood recirculating had increased. An urgent fistulagram was performed (Fig. 18.4).

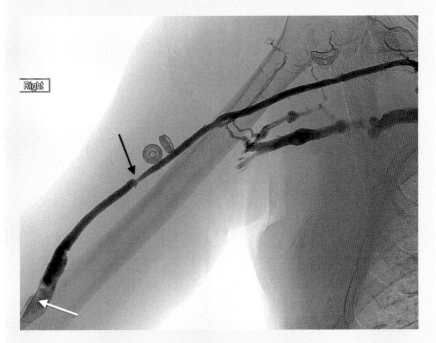

Fig. 18.4 A fistulagram study of the vein draining blood downstream from an arteriovenous fistula. The catheter can be seen in the fistula (*white arrow*). There is a tight stenosis in the cephalic vein (*black arrow*) related to a venous valve. The round objects next to the vein are fasteners on the patient's gown

The stenosis restricts the return of blood up the fistula towards the heart. During dialysis, a proportion of the blood flowing from the venous needle flows back to the arterial needle, recirculating around the dialyser (Fig. 18.5).

After the angioplasty (Fig 18.6), flow up the fistula was no longer restricted (Fig. 18.7).

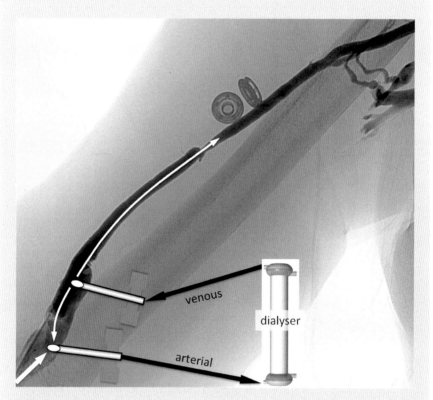

Fig. 18.5 Recirculation in the dialyser circuit. Blood is removed from the fistula vein via the arterial needle, pumped through the dialyser by the dialysis machine and returned to the fistula via the venous needle. The high resistance to flow up the fistula forces some of the returned blood back towards the arterial needle. It then flows round the dialyser circuit again

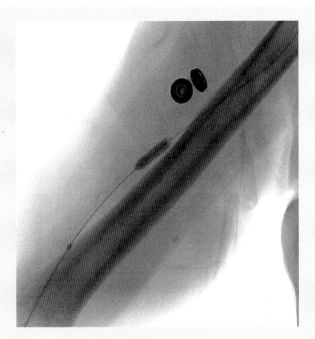

Fig. 18.6 Angioplasty balloon inflated at the site of the stenosis

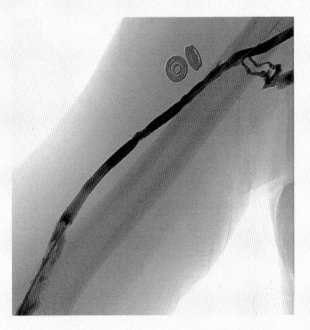

Fig. 18.7 Angiogram following angioplasty showing unobstructed flow up the fistula and through the cephalic vein

Complications of a Haemodialysis Catheter

The main complications of a haemodialysis catheter are infection, clotting and venous stenosis. Infection tends to track down the catheter from the exit site to form a biofilm around the catheter. This can lead to septicaemia, endocarditis and more distant seeding of infection such as osteomyelitis. Because of the serious consequences of infection, a dialysis catheter should not be used for any purpose other than dialysis.

Clotting of the catheter is detected when dialysis is attempted. Blood cannot be withdrawn if a clot or stenosis of the surrounding central vein obstructs flow.

If a catheter is in place for a prolonged period, stenosis and eventual occlusion of a central vein may occur. If an arteriovenous fistula is then created on the same side, the increase in venous pressure causes dilatation of veins over the upper chest and neck (Fig. 18.8).

Peritoneal Dialysis

In peritoneal dialysis, waste products are excreted by diffusion and convective flow across the peritoneal membrane into dialysis fluid in the peritoneal cavity. To achieve adequate dialysis, fluid needs to be exchanged every few hours, every day.

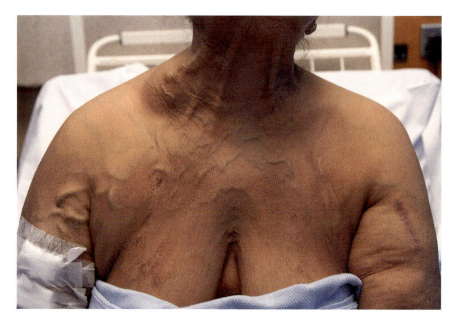

Fig. 18.8 Dilated veins across the right upper chest and neck of a lady due to occlusion of the right brachial vein in the axilla caused by a previous dialysis catheter. Venous blood flow is increased by an arteriovenous fistula in the right upper arm, covered with dressings. There are scars from a previous catheter and fistula surgery on her chest and left arm

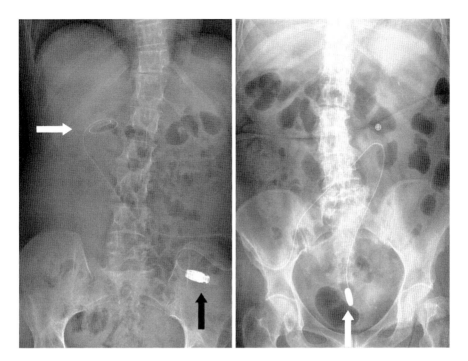

Fig. 18.9 Plain abdominal X-rays of two patients having peritoneal dialysis. The catheter on the left is malpositioned. Draining fluid in was slow and caused discomfort; fluid would not drain out. The curled end (*white arrow*) lies in the right upper quadrant under the liver. The radio-opaque tube connector (*black arrow*) is outside the body. The catheter on the right is correctly located. The radio-opaque weighted end of the catheter (*white arrow*) helps to keep it in the pelvic cavity

Fluid is drained in and out either manually (continuous ambulatory peritoneal dialysis, CAPD) or by a machine overnight (automated peritoneal dialysis, APD).

The catheter lying in the peritoneal cavity should allow dialysis fluid to flow freely in and out. If flow is slow or blocked, a plain abdominal X-ray is taken to check its position (Fig. 18.9).

Infection can affect the skin where the catheter emerges from abdomen (the 'exit site') (Fig. 18.10), the tunnel through the abdominal wall or the peritoneal fluid. PD peritonitis presents with abdominal pain and cloudy dialysis fluid but seldom leads to septicaemia.

Fluid Balance in a Dialysis Patient

With end-stage kidney failure, regulation of fluid balance is impaired. Many dialysis patients still have some residual kidney function and pass urine. However, the volume is often less than needed to maintain fluid balance.

Excess fluid is removed on haemodialysis by a hydrostatic pressure gradient across the dialyser membrane. In peritoneal dialysis, fluid is drawn into the

Fig. 18.10 Peritoneal catheter exit sites. (**a**) a healthy exit site – the skin around the catheter is dry and not inflamed. The dried exudate ('crusting') below the catheter does not indicate infection. The catheter is clean. (**b**) an unhealthy exit site – swollen granulation tissue is secreting purulent exudate and blood. There is dried material adherent to the catheter. A culture grew *Staphylococcus aureus*

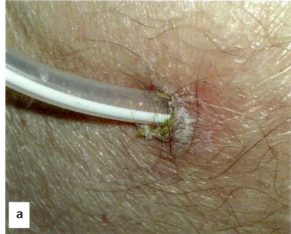

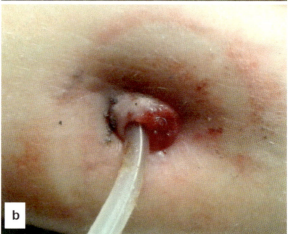

peritoneal cavity by an osmotic gradient created by glucose or other osmotic agent in the dialysis fluid.

It can be hard to judge fluid balance accurately from a clinical examination. Blood pressure may not be a reliable guide; it may be high due to the increased intravascular volume or low due to reduced left ventricular function despite fluid overload. Peripheral oedema may not be obvious, especially in younger patients. Techniques such as bioimpedance spectroscopy may give a more reliable estimate of fluid balance [3].

Measurement of changes in weight plays a key role in haemodialysis treatment. If urine and insensible losses together are less than the fluid in food and drink, the patient's body weight will increase between the end of one dialysis treatment and the start of the next. This is called the interdialytic weight gain. This fluid is removed

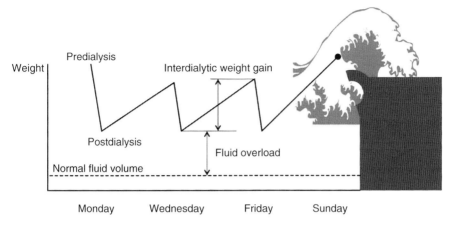

Fig. 18.11 The analogy of tide and waves

during the dialysis treatment by ultrafiltration. The rise and fall in weight across the week is like waves on the sea (Fig. 18.11).

Underneath the waves is the weight that the patient would have without kidney failure – the normal fluid volume. This weight rises and falls over a longer timescale as the patient loses and gains lean tissue mass during periods of acute illness and recovery. The difference between the post-dialysis weight and the normal fluid volume is the fluid overload.

Each dialysis patient has a prescribed target weight that should be reached by the end of each dialysis treatment. If the target weight is set lower than the patient's weight at normal fluid volume they may become hypotensive during dialysis – commonly called 'crashing'.

Conversely, if the target weight is not reduced after the patient has lost lean body mass there will be residual fluid overload. This is like a high tide underneath the waves. As the wave rises before the next treatment on top of the high tide, fluid may flood into the lungs (Fig. 18.12). This is more likely to happen at the weekend when there is a gap of 2 days rather than 1 between dialysis treatments.

Kidney Transplant

The most complete replacement of kidney function is achieved with a kidney transplant. Best results are obtained using kidneys donated by a live donor who is related to the recipient. Kidneys are otherwise obtained from deceased donors, either braindead or after the heart has stopped beating.

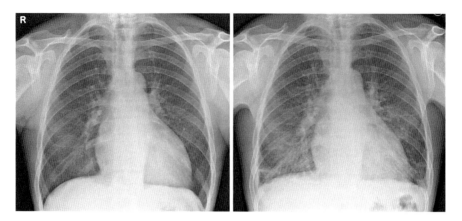

Fig. 18.12 Chest X-rays from a haemodialysis patient taken (*left*) when well and (*right*) when severely short of breath on arrival at the dialysis unit on a Monday. The right X-ray shows features of fluid overload with pulmonary vascular congestion, Kerley B lines and bilateral pleural effusions. The heart is enlarged on both X-rays

Detailed explanation of the transplant procedure and subsequent patient management are outside the scope of this book. We limit this section to problems that may present to a non-specialist clinician.

Causes of a Decline in Transplant Function

The likely cause of a decline in transplant kidney function changes with time after transplantation.

Acute kidney injury in the first week is usually due to:

- Hypovolaemia or acute tubular necrosis
- Hyperacute rejection
- Surgical problems with the blood supply or ureter

Declining function during the first 3 months is usually due to:

- Hypovolaemia
- Acute rejection – antibody or T cell-mediated
- Calcineurin inhibitor toxicity
- Interstitial nephritis
- Ureteric obstruction
- Recurrent focal segmental glomerulosclerosis (FSGS)
- Bacterial pyelonephritis
- BK virus infection

After 3 months, the following additional causes become increasingly common.

• Chronic rejection
• Chronic allograft nephropathy – interstitial fibrosis and tubular atrophy
• Non-adherence to immunosuppression
• Recurrent or de-novo glomerulonephritis
• Transplant artery stenosis

Immunosuppressive drugs prevent a decline in transplant function due to rejection but increase the risk of two other complications: infection and malignancy.

Infection

The type of infection that is most common varies over time after transplantation [4]:

• Within the first month, infections are usually due to environmental pathogens, such as catheter or wound infections and *Clostridium difficile* diarrhoea.
• Between 1 and 6 months, the type of infection depends upon the immunosuppressive treatment and whether the patient is taking prophylactic antimicrobial drugs. Cotrimoxazole is usually given to prevent *Pneumocystis jiroveci* pneumonia (PJP), formerly known as *Pneumocystis carinii* pneumonia (PCP). Antivirals such as valganciclovir may be given to prevent infection by herpes viruses such as cytomegalovirus (CMV).
• After the first 6 months, infections are more often due to conventional organisms such as community-acquired pneumonia and urinary tract infection. Late viral infections may appear, e.g., colitis or retinitis due to CMV, and herpes encephalitis (Patient 18.2). Opportunistic infections are commoner in patients who have had more intensive immunosuppression or particular environmental exposures such as to fungi.

Patient 18.2: Epstein-Barr Viral Encephalitis
Mr. Blackman had a kidney transplant in 2000. Ciclosporin and prednisolone were used for immunosuppression. The kidney did not function very well, eGFR was at best 25 ml/min/1.73 m^2. After 6 years, ciclosporin was substituted by mycophenolate mofetil to avoid calcineurin nephrotoxicity (see Sect. "Calcineurin inhibitors – two sides of a coin" in page 108).

Ten years after the transplant, he presented with a month's history of progressive difficulty swallowing solids and liquids, and hoarseness of his voice. He had lost 7 kg in weight.

He had been anticoagulated with warfarin for atrial fibrillation but during courses of antibiotics the INR was hard to control so had been stopped.

An MRI scan was reported as showing changes consistent with infarcts in the left cerebral hemisphere and the left side of the medulla (Fig. 18.13).

He was treated with aspirin and dipyridamole with a plan to restart warfarin, and required feeding via a nasogastric tube. Over the next 3 months his condition did not improve; his legs became weaker and his gait more unsteady. He was increasingly confused and so was readmitted to hospital.

A repeat MRI scan showed much more extensive white matter changes in the posterior fossa and cerebral hemispheres, consistent with encephalitis (Fig. 18.14).

His cerebrospinal fluid (CSF) contained 7 red blood cells per mm^3 and 139 white blood cells, of which 138 were lymphocytes. Epstein-Barr virus DNA (EBV, also called human herpesvirus 4 HHV-4) was detected in large amounts in the CSF (23,000 copies/ml). There was no EBV DNA in the blood but IgG against EBV was present, indicating previous infection

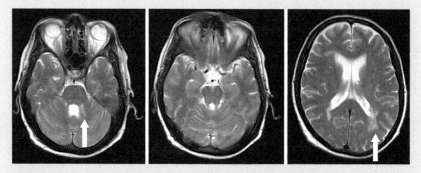

Fig. 18.13 MRI scan showing changes in the left side of the medulla and the left cerebral hemisphere (*arrows*)

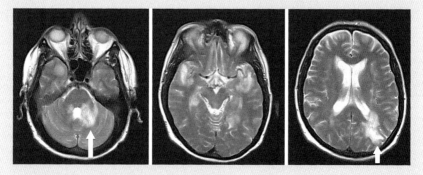

Fig. 18.14 MRI scan showing extensive white matter changes in the posterior fossa and cerebral hemispheres, consistent with encephalitis

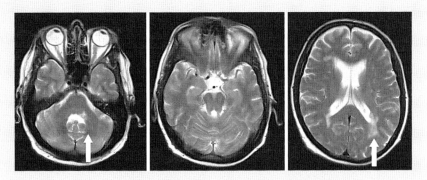

Fig. 18.15 MRI scan after 6 months showing improvement in the white matter changes

He was treated with 4 weeks of intravenous ganciclovir and then oral valganciclovir. Mycophenolate mofetil was stopped. Antiviral drugs were continued until EBV DNA was not detectable in the CSF. An MRI scan after 6 months showed marked improvement in the white matter changes (Fig. 18.15).

After a prolonged period of nasogastric feeding and intensive physiotherapy he made an excellent recovery.

After years of immunosuppression, warts caused by human papillomavirus can be very troublesome (Fig. 18.16). They are most common in patients treated with azathioprine [5] and may improve with reduction in the dose.

Malignancy

Long-term treatment with calcineurin inhibitors (tacrolimus and ciclosporin) may allow B cells infected with Epstein-Barr virus to proliferate, causing post-transplant lymphoproliferative disease (PTLD). Polyclonal PTLD may present with symptoms from the mass of lymph nodes, such as bowel obstruction. The nodes may regress if the immunosuppressants are stopped or reduced in dose [6]. Sometimes a clone of cells proliferates to become a monoclonal malignant lymphoma (Patient 18.3).

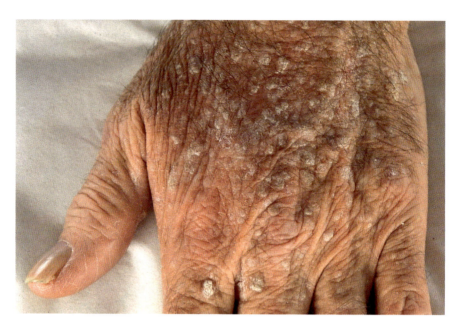

Fig. 18.16 Extensive warts on the hand of a kidney transplant patient who had taken prednisolone and azathioprine as immunosuppression for over 20 years

---

Patient 18.3: Post-transplant Lymphoproliferative Disease

Mr. Park's kidney transplant had functioned perfectly for 19 years, thanks to immunosuppression with prednisolone and ciclosporin. He developed symptoms of nausea and vomiting 1–2 h after meals and lost 4 kg in weight. A CT scan showed a stricture at the duodenal/jejunal flexure with thickening of the bowel wall (Fig. 18.17).

A biopsy of the thickened bowel showed high-grade diffuse large B cell lymphoma (non-germinal centre type). Further scans and a bone marrow trephine showed no sign of spread.

Ciclosporin was stopped and he was treated with R-CHOP chemotherapy – Rituximab, Cyclophosphamide, doxorubicin (Hydroxydaunomycin), vincristine (Oncovin®) and Prednisolone. His tumour regressed completely without perforation of the bowel wall, a complication that can result from tumour lysis.

A low dose of ciclosporin was restarted and prednisolone continued, but his transplant kidney function declined (Fig. 18.18).

A biopsy of the transplant kidney confirmed chronic rejection. He eventually restarted haemodialysis.

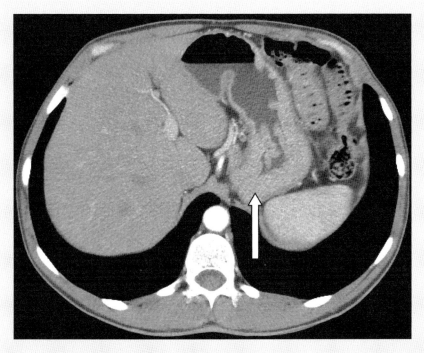

Fig. 18.17 Contrast CT scan showing thickening of the small bowel wall at the junction of the duodenum and jejunum (*arrow*) causing an obstruction to flow and fluid level in the dilated duodenum

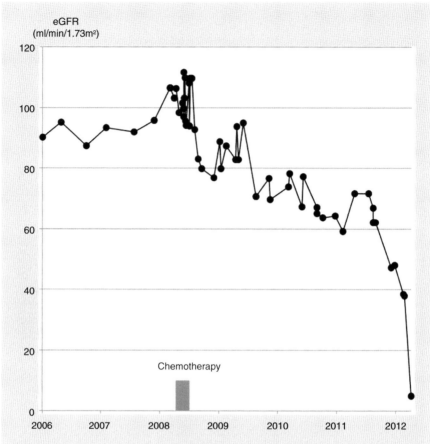

Fig. 18.18 Changes in kidney function after treatment for post-transplant lymphoprolif-erative disease

Long-term immunosuppression increases the risk of all forms of cancer. The commonest site is the skin, usually as a basal cell or squamous cell carcinoma (Figs. 18.19 and 18.20). Death from malignancy, such as lymphoma, lung or kidney cancer, is more common than in the general population [7].

**Figs. 18.19 and
18.20** Squamous cell
carcinoma on the scalp of a
kidney transplant patient

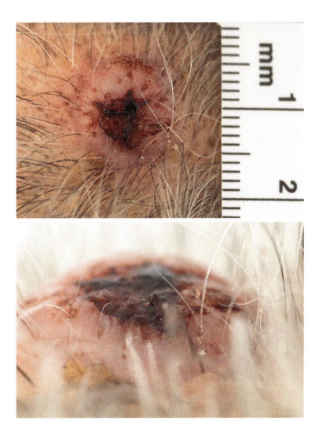

References

1. Siddiky A, Sarwar K, Ahmad N, Gilbert J. Management of arteriovenous fistulas. BMJ. 2014;349:g6262. doi:10.1136/bmj.g6262. http://www.bmj.com/content/349/bmj.g6262.
2. Zeraati A, Beladi Mousavi SS, Beladi MM. A review article: access recirculation among end stage renal disease patients undergoing maintenance hemodialysis. Nephrourol Mon. 2013;5(2):728–32. doi:10.5812/numonthly.6689. http://www.ncbi.nlm.nih.gov/pmc/articles/PMC3703129/.
3. Hecking M, Karaboyas A, Antlanger M, Saran R, Wizemann V, Chazot C, Rayner H, Hörl WH, Pisoni RL, Robinson BM, Sunder-Plassmann G, Moissl U, Kotanko P, Levin NW, Säemann MD, Kalantar-Zadeh K, Port FK, Wabel P. Significance of interdialytic weight gain versus chronic volume overload: consensus opinion. Am J Nephrol. 2013;38(1):78–90. doi:10.1159/000353104. Epub 2013 Jul 6. http://www.karger.com/Article/FullText/353104.
4. Karuthu S, Blumberg EA. Common infections in kidney transplant recipients. Clin J Am Soc Nephrol. 2012;7(12):2058–70. doi:10.2215/CJN.04410512. http://cjasn.asnjournals.org/content/7/12/2058.full.
5. Dicle O, Parmaksizoglu B, Gurkan A, Tuncer M, Demirbas A, Yilmaz E. Choice of immunosuppressants and the risk of warts in renal transplant recipients. Acta Derm Venereol. 2008;88(3):294–5. doi:10.2340/00015555-0411. http://www.medicaljournals.se/acta/content/?doi:10.2340/00015555-0411&html=1.

6. Starzl TE, Nalesnik MA, Porter KA, Ho M, Iwatsuki S, Griffith BP, Rosenthal JT, Hakala TR, Shaw Jr BW, Hardesty RL, Atchison RW, Jaffe R, Bahnson HT. Reversibility of lymphomas and lymphoproliferative lesions developing under cyclosporin-steroid therapy. Lancet. 1984;323(8377):583–7. http://www.ncbi.nlm.nih.gov/pmc/articles/PMC2987704/.
7. Farrugia D, Mahboob S, Cheshire J, Begaj I, Khosla S, Ray D, Sharif A. Malignancy-related mortality following kidney transplantation is common. Kidney Int. 2014;85(6):1395–403. doi:10.1038/ki.2013.458. http://www.nature.com/ki/journal/v85/n6/full/ki2013458a.html.

Chapter 19
Epilogue

Scaling-Up Kidney Care from One Individual to a Whole Population

Abstract In this chapter we explain:

- How one patient's experience changed a doctor's practice
- How to organise a community-wide kidney disease system
- How it is possible to reduce the prevalence of end-stage kidney failure

To complete this book, I (HR) would like to tell you a story. One morning in 2004, I was in the diabetes outpatient clinic. Before calling the next patient into the room, I reviewed his laboratory results. The serum creatinine was 204 micromol/L (2.3 mg/dL). At that time, 200 micromol/L prompted referral by the diabetes team to the nephrologist.

We were just starting to get used to using eGFR and I was surprised by how low it was in this patient – only 30 ml/min/1.73 m^2. I thought it would be interesting to draw a graph of his results. Figure 19.1 shows how it looked.

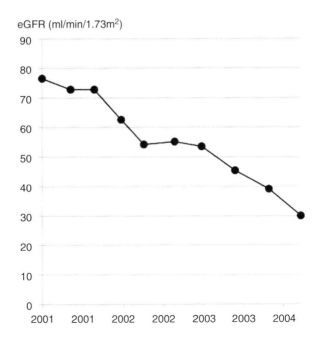

eGFR (ml/min/1.73m^2)

Fig. 19.1 Graph showing a linear decline in eGFR

© Springer International Publishing Switzerland 2016
H. Rayner et al., *Understanding Kidney Diseases*,
DOI 10.1007/978-3-319-23458-8_19

I was shocked to see that the latest eGFR was at the end of a linear trend that had been going on for years. This man's kidney failure was predictable but we had not predicted it. And to make matters worse, the patient was a doctor!

He was upset when I showed him the graph and unimpressed that I had not taken the trouble to work this out sooner. To add to my humiliation, he asked for a second opinion. Since then, I have drawn an eGFR graph for pretty much every kidney patient I see.

A few days later, my bank telephoned me to enquire about suspicious transactions on my credit card. It turned out to be a false alarm. When I asked how their suspicions had been raised, the clerk explained that the bank's computer had alerted them to unusual patterns of transactions on my account. From her tone of voice, she seemed surprised I was not already aware of this service!

If the bank was using simple computer rules to take care of my money, shouldn't I do the same to find patients whose kidney function was behaving suspiciously? I decided to use a register of all the kidney and diabetes patients who had attended the hospital to find patients whose eGFR graph suggested they were heading for trouble.

Every week since then I have reviewed the graphs of patients with diabetes who have a new eGFR result. For the details of this system, please take a look at our report [1]. The system has meant that patients come to the specialist clinic at an earlier stage of kidney disease, giving more opportunity to improve their kidney function and to prepare them properly for a transplant or dialysis.

The eGFR graph system allows me to follow up patients' kidney function while their Primary Care team is monitoring it. Patients with a stable eGFR (see Sect. "Analysing variation in eGFR" in page 34) no longer need to attend the clinic in person. This is very popular with patients and with me!

Building on the success of this system, our pathology laboratory now provides a similar monitoring service for all eGFR tests requested by Primary Care clinicians [2].

For more details of this integrated system of care, please have a look at our report [3].

After working in this way for over ten years, the number of patients having dialysis in our community is going down (Fig. 19.2) – the opposite of the trend in the rest of England.

Fig. 19.2 The prevalent number of patients receiving dialysis or with a functioning kidney transplant each month under the care of the Heart of England NHS Foundation Trust

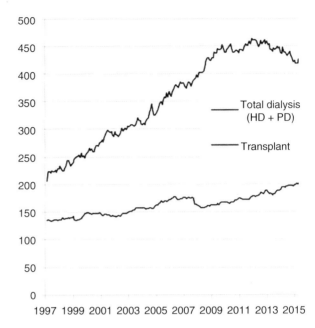

References

1. Rayner HC, Hollingworth L, Higgins R, Dodds S. Systematic kidney disease management in a population with diabetes mellitus: turning the tide of kidney failure. BMJ Qual Saf. 2011. doi:10.1136/bmjqs-2011-000061. http://qualitysafety.bmj.com/content/20/10/903.abstract.
2. Kennedy DM, Chatha K, Rayner HC. Laboratory database population surveillance to improve detection of progressive chronic kidney disease. J Renal Care. 2013;39 Suppl 2:23–9. doi:10.1111/j.1755-6686.2013.12029.x. http://onlinelibrary.wiley.com/doi/10.1111/j.1755-6686.2013.12029.x/pdf.
3. Rayner HC, Baharani J, Dasgupta I, Suresh V, Temple RM, Thomas ME, Smith SA. Does community-wide chronic kidney disease management improve patient outcomes? Nephrol Dial Transplant. 2014;29(3):644–9. doi:10.1093/ndt/gft486. http://ndt.oxfordjournals.org/content/29/3/644.abstract.

Multiple Choice Questions

Chapter 1

1. At what rate does the GFR typically decline in males after the age of 45 years?

   (a) 0.1 ml/min/1.73 m^2
   (b) 0.5 ml/min/1.73 m^2
   (c) 0.8 ml/min/1.73 m^2
   (d) 1.2 ml/min/1.73 m^2
   (e) 2 ml/min/1.73 m^2

2. Which of the following does not form part of the glomerular filtration barrier?

   (a) Endothelial cell fenestration
   (b) Sub-endothelial space
   (c) Glomerular basement membrane
   (d) Podocyte foot process slit diaphragm
   (e) Sub-podocyte space

3. Which of the following cell types does not perform a phagocytic function?

   (a) Glomerular endothelial cell
   (b) Mesangial cell
   (c) Macrophage
   (d) Podocyte
   (e) Proximal tubular epithelial cell

4. Which of the following statements about angiotensin II is false?

   (a) It causes vasoconstriction of the efferent arteriole
   (b) It increases the amount of albumin filtered by the glomeruli
   (c) It is increased in renal acidosis
   (d) It increases aldosterone production
   (e) It is reduced in people with diabetes

© Springer International Publishing Switzerland 2016
H. Rayner et al., *Understanding Kidney Diseases*,
DOI 10.1007/978-3-319-23458-8

Chapter 2

5. Which of the following does not affect the serum creatinine concentration in chronic kidney disease?

   (a) Glomerular filtration rate
   (b) Tubular secretory function
   (c) Fluid overload
   (d) Skeletal muscle mass
   (e) Ethnic origin

6. Which of the following is not required to estimate GFR using the MDRD equation?

   (a) Age
   (b) Sex
   (c) Race
   (d) Creatinine
   (e) Body weight

7. In which of the following circumstances is the urea-to-creatinine ratio most likely to increase?

   (a) A malnourished patient with small muscle mass
   (b) A bodybuilder taking protein supplements
   (c) High blood pressure treated with vasodilator drugs
   (d) When the rate of flow of filtrate along the nephron is slowed
   (e) Trimethoprim therapy

Chapter 3

8. Which of the following indicates that a series of data points is not stable?

   (a) The mean is decreasing slowly over time
   (b) The control limits lie outside the data points
   (c) Three consecutive points are below the mean
   (d) Three consecutive points are in a decline
   (e) The mean is greater than the median

9. After unilateral nephrectomy, how long does it take the serum creatinine concentration to reach a new equilibrium?

   (a) 6 h
   (b) 12 h
   (c) 24 h
   (d) 48 h
   (e) 72 h

10. An adult male who normally has a serum creatinine of 120 micromol/L (1.4 mg/dL) presents to hospital with a serum creatinine of 320 micromol/L (3.6 mg/dL). According to the Kidney Disease Improving Global Outcomes (KDIGO), what stage of acute kidney injury has been reached?

   (a) Stage 1
   (b) Stage 2
   (c) Stage 3
   (d) Stage 4
   (e) Stage 5

Chapter 4

11. At a routine checkup, a 42-year-old male with diabetes is found to have an eGFR of 32 ml/min/1.73 m^2. When repeated 3 months later, it is 35 ml/min/1.73 m^2. His albumin:creatinine ratio (ACR) is 35 mg/mmol (310 mg/g). Macroalbuminuria is defined as ACR >30 mg/mmol (>300 mg/g). What stage of CKD does he have?

   (a) Stage G4A2
   (b) Stage G2A1
   (c) Stage G4A3
   (d) Stage G3A3
   (e) Stage G3A2

12. Which of the following is not a typical symptom of kidney failure?

   (a) Insomnia
   (b) Hallucinations
   (c) Itching
   (d) Restless legs
   (e) Nausea

Chapter 5

13. In a patient with diabetic nephropathy and proteinuria, which of the following is not associated with the rate of decline in GFR?

   (a) Glycated haemoglobin (HbA1c) concentration
   (b) Mean arterial pressure
   (c) Serum bicarbonate
   (d) Serum total CO_2
   (e) Urinary angiotensinogen

14. Which of the following is an indication for renal artery angioplasty?

   (a) Systolic blood pressure >240 mmHg
   (b) Flash pulmonary oedema
   (c) eGFR <30 ml/min/1.73 m^2
   (d) Decline in eGFR of >10 ml/min/1.73 m^2/year
   (e) Blood pressure requiring >3 different antihypertensives

15. Which of the following is not a typical feature of cholesterol crystal embolisation?

    (a) Elevated CRP
    (b) Eosinophilia
    (c) Peripheral vascular atherosclerosis
    (d) Positive ANA
    (e) Decline in eGFR over weeks

Chapter 6

16. Which of the following is not associated with an increased risk of pre-eclampsia?

    (a) Fourth pregnancy
    (b) New paternity
    (c) Multiple pregnancy
    (d) Obesity
    (e) Chronic kidney disease

17. Which of the following is not associated with chronic kidney disease?

    (a) Polyhydramnios
    (b) Intrauterine growth retardation
    (c) Premature delivery
    (d) Down's syndrome
    (e) Spontaneous abortion

Chapter 7

18. Which of the following is not a feature of Alport syndrome?

    (a) Deafness
    (b) Visual impairment
    (c) Proteinuria
    (d) Microscopic haematuria
    (e) Renal failure

19. Polycystic kidney disease is thought to be primarily due to a genetic abnormality of:

    (a) Sodium transport
    (b) Cell division
    (c) Tubular membrane structure
    (d) Epithelial permeability
    (e) Cilial function

20. Which of the following is not an inherited disease affecting nephron function?

    (a) Von Hippel Lindau syndrome
    (b) Gitelman syndrome
    (c) Liddle syndrome
    (d) Bartter syndrome
    (e) Dent disease

21. Furosemide acts on which part of the nephron?

    (a) Proximal tubule
    (b) Descending limb of the loop of Henle
    (c) Ascending limb of the loop of Henle
    (d) Distal tubule
    (e) Collecting duct

Chapter 8

22. An 80-year-old lady was prescribed ramipril 10 mg daily. Which of the following suggests this drug was adversely affecting her kidney function?

    (a) High urea-to-creatinine ratio
    (b) eGFR <15 ml/min/1.73 m^2
    (c) Systolic blood pressure <110 mmHg
    (d) An irritating dry cough
    (e) Hypokalaemia

23. Which of the following drugs is a common cause of interstitial nephritis?

    (a) Metformin
    (b) Ranitidine
    (c) Lithium
    (d) Omeprazole
    (e) Ondansetron

24. Which of the following is not nephrotoxic?

    (a) Gentamicin
    (b) Cadmium
    (c) Metformin
    (d) Lithium
    (e) Orellanine

Chapter 9

25. Which of the following is not associated with impaired growth in children?

    (a) Congenital nephrotic syndrome
    (b) Vesico-ureteric reflux
    (c) Autosomal recessive polycystic kidney disease
    (d) Steroid therapy
    (e) Social deprivation

26. Which of the following statements about obesity is false?

    (a) It is associated with proteinuria
    (b) Weight loss reduces the risk of kidney disease in people with diabetes
    (c) In increases the risk of complications after transplant surgery
    (d) It increases the risk of mortality in dialysis patients
    (e) It is associated with hypertension

Chapter 10

27. Which of the following statements about hypertension is false?

    (a) Antihypertensive medication is better taken before bed
    (b) Nocturnal hypertension is more common in CKD
    (c) The arm with the lower blood pressure is used
    (d) Patient self-management improves control of blood pressure
    (e) High blood pressure increases the risk of end-stage kidney disease

Chapter 11

28. In IgA nephropathy, which of the following does not indicate an increased risk of renal failure?

    (a) Proteinuria
    (b) High blood pressure
    (c) Reduced glomerular filtration rate
    (d) Interstitial fibrosis on kidney biopsy
    (e) Macroscopic haematuria

29. Which of the following statements about myoglobin is false?

    (a) It is freely filtered by glomeruli
    (b) It is glomerulotoxic
    (c) It is reabsorbed by the proximal tubule
    (d) It colours urine dark red
    (e) It is detected by the urine dipstick test for blood

30. Which of the following is not a feature of the nephrotic syndrome?

    (a) Proteinuria greater than 5 g/ day
    (b) Hypercholesterolaemia
    (c) Microscopic haematuria
    (d) Peripheral oedema
    (e) Hypoalbuminaemia

31. Who of the following should be treated with antibiotics?

    (a) A man with a urinary catheter and a positive urine culture
    (b) A woman with diabetes and a positive urine culture from a mid-stream urine specimen
    (c) A man with a culture of 104 CFU/ml from a mid-stream urine specimen
    (d) A woman with frequency, dysuria, fever and a negative urine culture
    (e) A man with a positive dipstick test for nitrites and leucocytes

Chapter 12

32. Which of the following statements is correct?

    (a) Raised jugular venous pressure is a reliable marker of fluid overload
    (b) High blood pressure indicates increased total body sodium
    (c) Increased total body sodium usually causes high blood pressure
    (d) Lymphoedema is incompressible
    (e) Sleeping in a chair worsens leg oedema

33. Which of the following statements about a vasculitic rash is false?

    (a) It is found on the legs in Henoch-Schönlein purpura
    (b) It blanches when compressed
    (c) It may cause necrotic ulcers
    (d) IgA is deposited in the skin in Henoch-Schönlein purpura
    (e) Blood and protein in the urine means urgent referral is required

Chapter 13

34. Which of the following statements about erythropoietin production in an adult is true?

    (a) It is divided between the liver and the kidneys
    (b) It is inhibited by NSAIDs
    (c) It is stimulated by muscle hypoxia
    (d) It is located in the interstitial cells
    (e) It is down-regulated in chronic kidney disease

35. Which of the following statements about treatment of renal acidosis is false?

    (a) Fruit and vegetable diet is effective
    (b) Sodium bicarbonate lowers angiotensin production in the kidney
    (c) Sodium bicarbonate reduces the rate of decline in GFR
    (d) Sodium bicarbonate increases muscle mass
    (e) Sodium bicarbonate causes high blood pressure

36. Which of the following statements about parathyroid hormone synthesis is true?

    (a) It is stimulated by hypocalcaemia
    (b) It is stimulated by activated vitamin D3
    (c) It is inhibited by hyperphosphataemia
    (d) It is stimulated by FGF-23
    (e) It is autonomous in secondary hyperparathyroidism

37. Which of the following statements about hypercalcaemia is false?

    (a) It reduces GFR due to vasoconstriction
    (b) It impairs urinary concentration
    (c) It can be caused by loop diuretics
    (d) It is associated with raised alkaline phosphatase with metastatic carcinoma
    (e) It is associated with normal alkaline phosphatase in multiple myeloma

Chapter 14

38. Which of the following statements about myeloma is false?

    (a) Free light chains are filtered by glomeruli
    (b) Free light chains form casts with uromodulin
    (c) Bence Jones proteinuria is not detected by urine protein dipsticks
    (d) Renal function can recover with chemotherapy treatment
    (e) A significantly raised concentration of serum free light chains is diagnostic

39. Which of the following statements about amyloid is false?

    (a) It develops in the skeleton of some patients in the first 5 years of dialysis
    (b) When deposited in the kidney, it causes proteinuria
    (c) It is shown by Congo red staining on histology
    (d) It is composed of proteins arranged in a beta-pleated sheet
    (e) Chronic inflammation causes AA type amyloid

40. Which of the following antibody is found in post-streptococcal glomerulonephritis?

    (a) anti-streptolysin B
    (b) anti-DNAse B
    (c) anti-hyaluronic acid
    (d) anti-staphylokinase
    (e) anti-adenine dinucleotidase

41. Which of the following statements about ANCA-associated vasculitis is true?

    (a) C-ANCA is associated with microscopic polyangiitis
    (b) MPO-ANCA is usually C-ANCA
    (c) PR3-ANCA is usually C-ANCA
    (d) A rising titre of MPO-ANCA indicates a need to increase immunosuppression
    (e) ANCA-associated vasculitis is usually cured by a prolonged course of cyclophosphamide

Chapter 15

42. Which of the following is the modality of choice for detecting renal stones?

    (a) Ultrasound
    (b) Doppler ultrasound
    (c) Isotope renography
    (d) CT scanning
    (e) MRI scanning

43. Which of the following statements about contrast-induced nephropathy is true?

    (a) It can be ameliorated by sodium chloride infusion before the procedure
    (b) It often requires temporary dialysis
    (c) It is commoner in women
    (d) It is less likely with hyper-osmolar contrast medium
    (e) Is it rare if the eGFR is >30 ml/min/1.73 m^2

Chapter 16

44. Which of the following statements about kidney biopsy is true?

    (a) It is usually required to confirm a diagnosis of diabetic nephropathy
    (b) It causes bleeding in a minority of patients
    (c) It is essential to diagnose anti-glomerular basement membrane disease
    (d) It requires a general anaesthetic
    (e) It should only be performed if it will change patient management

Chapter 17

45. In someone aged 35 years with an eGFR of 65 ml/min/1.73 m^2, by how much does an albumin:creatinine ratio of 42 mg/mmol increase the risk of mortality compared to no albuminuria?

    (a) 1.5 times
    (b) 2 times
    (c) 4 times
    (d) 9 times
    (e) 12 times

46. When should a patient be transferred to the multidisciplinary team to prepare them for dialysis?

    (a) When the eGFR goes below 20 ml/min/1.73 m^2
    (b) When the patient develops symptoms of uraemia
    (c) When the eGFR goes below 10 ml/min/1.73 m^2
    (d) When the rate of decline in eGFR is greater than 10 ml/min/1.73 m^2/year
    (e) When dialysis is likely to be needed within the next 12 months

47. Which of the following statements about renal replacement therapy is true?

    (a) It is unethical not to treat someone with dialysis with an eGFR less than 5 ml/min/1.73 m^2
    (b) Mortality is less with a kidney transplant than dialysis
    (c) Mortality is less with peritoneal dialysis than haemodialysis
    (d) The minimum frequency of haemodialysis is three times per week
    (e) Peritoneal dialysis is done 5 days per week

Chapter 18

48. Which of the following statements about an arterio-venous fistula is true?

    (a) It is contraindicated if the left ventricular ejection fraction is less than 40 %
    (b) The blood flow is good if it remains full of blood when the arm is elevated
    (c) The thrill should only be felt in systole
    (d) The dialysis needle is inserted as near to the anastomosis as possible
    (e) The risk of infection is lower than with a dialysis catheter

49. Which of the following statements about a peritoneal dialysis catheter is true?

    (a) Fluid should take under 20 min to drain out
    (b) The tip should be located in the centre of the abdomen
    (c) Fluid should be slightly cloudy on draining out
    (d) Dried exudate ('crusting') at the exit site should be treated with antibiotics
    (e) It should be replaced once a year to reduce the risk of infection

50. Which of the following statements about a kidney transplant patient is false?

    (a) Infections after 12 months are usually due to conventional organisms
    (b) Post-transplant lymphoproliferative disease is due to T cell proliferation
    (c) Cotrimoxazole is used to prevent *Pneumocystis jiroveci* pneumonia (PJP)
    (d) The commonest site of malignancy is the skin
    (e) Post-transplant lymphoproliferative disease may regress if immunosuppressive drugs are stopped

Multiple Choice Question Answers

Question	Answer
1.	(d)
2.	(b)
3.	(a)
4.	(e)
5.	(c)
6.	(e)
7.	(d)
8.	(a)
9.	(b)
10.	(c)
11.	(d)
12.	(b)
13.	(a)
14.	(b)
15.	(d)
16.	(a)
17.	(d)
18.	(b)
19.	(e)
20.	(a)
21.	(c)
22.	(a)
23.	(d)
24.	(c)
25.	(b)
26.	(d)
27.	(c)
28	(e)
29.	(b)
30.	(c)

© Springer International Publishing Switzerland 2016
H. Rayner et al., *Understanding Kidney Diseases*,
DOI 10.1007/978-3-319-23458-8

Question	Answer
31.	(d)
32.	(e)
33.	(b)
34.	(d)
35.	(e)
36.	(a)
37.	(c)
38.	(e)
39.	(a)
40.	(b)
41.	(c)
42.	(d)
43.	(a)
44.	(e)
45.	(c)
46.	(e)
47.	(b)
48.	(e)
49.	(a)
50.	(b)

Index of Case Reports

ACE inhibitor nephrotoxicity	8.1, 8.3, 11.6
Acute kidney injury	3.2, 8.1, 8.2, 8.3, 11.6, 12.1, 13.2, 13.3, 13.7, 13.8, 14.1, 15.1, 15.5, 16.1
Anaemia	13.1
Atherosclerosis	5.3
Cervical carcinoma	11.7
Cholesterol crystal embolisation	5.3
Chronic kidney disease	2.1, 2.2, 8.4, 9.2, 9.4, 10.1, 13.1, 13.4, 13.5, 13.6, 17.1, 17.2
Crescentic glomerulonephritis	16.1
Diabetic nephropathy	3.1, 3.3, 5.1, 5.2, 8.1, 10.1, 17.2
End-stage kidney disease	4.2, 17.2, 17.3
Epstein-Barr viral encephalitis	18.2
Haemodialysis	18.1
Haemolytic uraemic syndrome	13.2, 13.3
Hypercalcaemia	13.7, 13.8
Hyperparathyroidism	13.5, 13.6
IgA nephropathy	11.2, 11.3, 11.4
Interstitial nephritis	16.2
Lithium nephrotoxicity	8.4
Malignancy	13.7
Multiple myeloma	14.1
Nephrotic syndrome	5.2, 9.1, 9.3
Nephrotoxicity, ACE inhibitor	8.1, 8.3, 11.6
Nephrotoxicity, lithium	8.4
Nephrotoxicity, NSAID	8.2
Normal kidneys with low eGFR	2.3
Obstructive uropathy	3.4, 11.7
Parathyroidectomy	13.6
Post-transplant lymphoproliferative disease	18.3
Pre-eclampsia	6.1

© Springer International Publishing Switzerland 2016
H. Rayner et al., *Understanding Kidney Diseases*,
DOI 10.1007/978-3-319-23458-8

Pruritus	4.1
Puberty	9.4
Renal bone disease	9.2, 9.4, 13.4
Retroperitoneal fibrosis	15.1
Rhabdomyolysis	11.5
Sarcoidosis	13.8
Sepsis	3.2, 12.1
Thin glomerular basement membrane disease	11.1
Transplant kidney	2.4, 9.2, 9.4, 18.2, 18.3
Trimethoprim effect	2.4
Urinary infection	11.7
Uromodulin kidney disease	7.1
Vasculitis	14.2, 14.3
Vesico-ureteric reflux	6.1, 7.2

Index of Histopathology, Radiology and Clinical Images

Pathology	Figure
Alport syndrome	7.1
Amyloidosis	14.2–14.3
Anti-GBM disease	14.10
Arterio-venous fistula	18.3–18.7
Autosomal dominant polycystic kidney disease	7.6, 7.7, 15.6
Calcineurin (ciclosporin) nephrotoxicity	8.4
Carcinoma cervix	11.25–11.27
Central venous thrombosis	18.8
Cholesterol crystal embolism	5.13, 5.15
Chronic kidney disease	15.3
Crescentic glomerulonephritis	14.7
Cutaneous vasculitis	12.6, 12.7, 12.8
Cyst	15.5
Diabetic nephropathy	5.6, 5.7, 11.14
EBV encephalitis	18.13–18.15
Emphysematous pyelonephritis	15.22
Henoch-Schoenlein purpura	12.5
Hyperparathyroidism	13.8–13.11
IgA nephropathy	11.5, 11.6, 11.9
Interstitial nephritis	8.7, 16.3
Kidney scar	15.4
Membranous nephropathy	14.11–14.13
Metastatic carcinoma	13.13–13.14
Microangiopathic haemolytic anaemia	13.3
Minimal change nephrotic syndrome	11.19
Myoglobinuria	11.12
Necrotising vasculitis	14.6
Nephrotic syndrome	11.18, 12.2
Normal kidney	1.4, 1.5, 1.6, 15.1, 15.2, 15.15, 15.23, 16.1
Obstructive uropathy	11.22–11.27, 12.9, 15.7–15.9

© Springer International Publishing Switzerland 2016
H. Rayner et al., *Understanding Kidney Diseases*,
DOI 10.1007/978-3-319-23458-8

Pathology	Figure
Peritoneal dialysis catheter	18.9, 18.10
Post-streptococcal glomerulonephritis	14.5
Post-transplant lymphoproliferative disease	18.17
Pulmonary oedema	18.12
Renal artery stenosis	5.9, 5.10, 5.12
Renal infarction	15.24
Retroperitoneal fibrosis	15.10–15.14
Sarcoidosis	13.15–13.17
Squamous cell carcinoma	18.19, 18.20
Steal syndrome	18.2
Thin glomerular basement membrane disease	11.4
Thrombotic microangiopathy	13.4
Uraemic pruritus	4.3, 4.4
Ureteric stone	15.20, 15.21
Ureteric tumour	15.16–15.19
Vesico-ureteric reflux	7.8–7.13
Warts	18.16

Index

A

ACE inhibitor, 109
Acid–base balance, 180
Acquired cystic disease, 216
ACR. *See* Albumin:creatinine ratio (ACR)
Acute inflammation, 164
Acute kidney injury, 42–44, 114, 142, 146, 151, 164
Acute-phase reactant, 149
ADAMTS13, 179
ADPKD. *See* Polycystic kidney disease:autosomal dominant (ADPKD)
AHase. *See* Anti-hyaluronidase (AHase)
Albumin:creatinine ratio (ACR), 144, 237
Aldosterone, 89, 105
Alkaline phosphatase, 187
1-Alpha-hydroxylase, 183
Alport syndrome, 84
Alternative remedies, 103
Alveolar haemorrhage, 210
Aminoglycoside antibiotics, 112
Ammonium ions (NH_4^+), 180
Amyloid fibrils, 202
Amyloidosis, 73, 198, 200
Anaemia, 173
Analbuminaemia, 149
Analysing variation, 34–38
ANCA. *See* Anti-neutrophil cytoplasmic antibody (ANCA)
Angioplasty, 68
Angiotensin converting enzyme, 190
Angiotensin converting enzyme (ACE) inhibitors, 105
Angiotensin-II (A-II), 3, 104

Angiotensinogen, 181
Angiotensin Receptor Blockers (ARBs), 105
Anterior lenticonus, 84
Antidiuretic hormone, 89
Anti-DNAse B antibodies, 204
Anti-dsDNA antibody, 202
Anti-glomerular basement membrane antibody (anti-GBM ab), 210
Anti-hyaluronidase (AHase), 204
Anti-myeloperoxidase (MPO), 204
Anti-neutrophil cytoplasmic antibody (ANCA), 204
Anti-nicotinamide-adenine dinucleotidase (anti-NAD), 204
Anti-nuclear antibody, 202
Anti-phospholipase A_2 receptor antibody (anti-PLA$_2$R ab), 211
Anti-proteinase 3 (PR3), 204
Anti-streptokinase (ASKase), 204
Anti-streptolysin O (ASO), 204
Antithrombin III, 151
Apolipoproteins, 149
Aquaporin 2, 89
Arterioles:efferent, 104
Arteriovenous (AV) fistula, 176, 255
Art lessons, 250
Aspirin, 79
Atherosclerosis, 67
Atypical haemolytic uraemic syndrome (aHUS), 84, 203
Automated peritoneal dialysis, APD, 263
Autoregulation, 3, 129
Autosomal dominant polycystic kidney disease (ADPKD), 16

© Springer International Publishing Switzerland 2016
H. Rayner et al., *Understanding Kidney Diseases*,
DOI 10.1007/978-3-319-23458-8

B

Bacterial endocarditis glomerulonephritis, 203
Bacteriuria, asymptomatic, 152
Bardet-Biedl syndrome, 92
Bartter syndrome, 86
Basal cell carcinoma, 272
Berry aneurysms, 94
Bicarbonate, 180
Bioimpedance spectroscopy, 264
Bipolar disorder, 110
BK virus, 266
Bone maturation, 122
Bosniak classification, 216
British Kidney Patient Association, 251
BUN-to-creatinine ratio, 26, 105, 164

C

Cadmium, 114
CAKUT, 95
Calcineurin inhibitors, 108, 266
Calcitriol, 183
Cancer, 272
Casts, 135, 142
    nephropathy, 199
C3 glomerulopathy, 203
Cholesterol, 149
Cholesterol crystal embolism, 71–73, 203
Chronic allograft nephropathy, 267
Chronic kidney disease, 129
Chronic retention of urine, 170
Ciclosporin, 108
Cilia, 92
CIN. See Contrast-induced nephropathy (CIN)
Cinacalcet, 186
CKD-EPI equation, 15
CKD progression, 145
Cocaine, 113
Coeliac disease, 176
Colony Forming Units, 152
Complement, 177, 179, 202
Congenital nephrotic syndrome, 84–86, 117
Congo red, 201
Conservative care, 249
Continuous ambulatory peritoneal dialysis
        (CAPD), 263
Contrast-induced nephropathy (CIN), 227–228
Control limits, 35
Cortical scar, 217
Cortico-medullary differentiation, 215
'Crashing,' 265
Creatinine, 11, 23
Crescentic glomerulonephritis, 234
Cryoglobulinaemia, 203

Cryoglobulins, 74
CT urogram, 226
Cyclo-oxygenase enzymes, 107
Cystatin C, 24
Cysteine stones, 88
Cystic kidney diseases, 91
Cystinuria, 88
Cysts, 215
Cytomegalovirus (CMV), 267

D

DBP. See Vitamin D-binding protein (DBP)
Dense Deposit Disease, 203
Dent type 1 disease, 88
Depression, 250
Diabetes, 275
    insipidus, 110
        nephrogenic, 89
    mellitus, 59–67, 109, 144
        glucose control, 61
        nephropathy, 59
Diabetic nephropathy, 130, 146, 150, 232
Dialysis, 243, 277
    amyloidosis, 200
    starting, 249
Diuretic, 109, 149, 163
    amiloride, 89, 110
    furosemide, 86, 87
    loop, 86
    potassium sparing, 89
    spironolactone, 87
    thiazide, 89
Diurnal rhythm, 126
DMSA scan, 96
Dronedarone, 25

E

Eculizumab, 177, 179
eGFR, 13
Emphysematous pyelonephritis, 227
Enterococcus faecalis, 154
Eosinophils, 113
Erythroid progenitor cells, 173
Erythropoietin, 173
Escherichia coli subtype O157, 177
Ethylene glycol, 114
Exercise, 250

F

Fanconi syndrome, 88, 184
Fatigue, 52

FGF-23. *See* Fibroblast growth factor 23 (FGF-23)
Fibrinoid necrosis, 206
Fibroblast growth factor 23 (FGF-23), 183
Fibrocystin/polyductin, 92
Fibromuscular dysplasia, 69
Fluid balance, 161
Fluid overload, 264
Fluid restriction, 163
Foamy urine, 143
Focal segmental glomerulosclerosis (FSGS), 74, 83, 123, 266
Free light chains, 198
Fruits and vegetables, 181

G
Gabapentin, 53
Gadolinium, 229
Gentamicin, 112
Gitelman syndrome, 89
Glomerular filtration, 1
    barrier, 85, 143
    pressure, 105
Glomerular filtration rate (GFR), 7, 11
Glomerulonephritis, 113
Glomerulonephritis, proliferative, 204
Glomerulosclerosis, 129
Glomerulus
    number, 7
    size, 7
Glyphosate, 114
Goodpasture's syndrome, 210
Gordon's syndrome, 89
Gout, 90
Growth
    hormone, 119
    pubertal spurt, 122
    retardation, 119

H
Haematuria, 134, 204
Haemodialysis, 176, 249, 265
Haemodialysis:disequilibrium, 55
Haemoglobin, regulatory mechanism, 176
Haemoglobinuria, 134
Haemolytic uraemic syndrome (HUS)
    atypical, 177
    diarrhoea-positive, 177
Head circumference, 117
Height, 117
Henoch-Schönlein Purpura, 168
Hepatitis B, 73, 114

Hepatitis C, 73, 114
Hereditary nephritis, 84
Heroin, 113–114
Herpes encephalitis, 267
HIF. *See* Hypoxia-inducible factor (HIF)
High blood pressure, 61
HIV, 114
HIV-associated nephropathy (HIVAN), 74
Hungry bone syndrome, 187
HUS. *See* Haemolytic uraemic syndrome (HUS)
Hydronephrosis, 220
Hydroureter, 225
Hypercalcaemia, 142, 189
Hyperfiltration, 78, 96
Hyperparathyroidism, 110, 183, 184
Hypocalcaemia, 142
Hypoxia-inducible factor (HIF), 174

I
Immunoglobulin A (IgA) nephropathy, 137, 198, 204
Immunoglobulins, 198
Indoxyl sulfate, 240
Insomnia, 52
Insulin-like growth factor 1 (IGF-1), 119
Integrated care, 272
Intercalated cells, 89
Interdialytic weight gain, 264
Interstitial cells, 174
Interstitial nephritis, 112–114, 233
Ischaemic polyneuropathy, 257
Ischaemic preconditioning, 110
Isotope renography, 223
Itching, 52

K
Kidney
    biopsy, 231
    blood flow, 7
    donor, 240
    transplant, 108, 120, 123, 255
    tumours, 94
Klotho, 240

L
Lactate dehydrogenase (LDH), 176
Lactic acidosis, 113
Laminin, 85
LDH. *See* Lactate dehydrogenase (LDH)
Lead, 114

Letters to patients, 248
Leucocytes, 154
Leucocytoclastic vasculitis, 169
Liddle syndrome, 89
Lithium, 110–112
Loop of Henle, 86
Lymphoedema, 162

M
Macroalbuminuria, 145
Macula densa, 4, 112
Magnetic resonance imaging, 229
MAG3 renogram, 96, 223
MAHA. *See* Microangiopathic haemolytic
        anaemia (MAHA)
Malignancy, 190
Malignant hypertension, 114, 131
Malignant lymphoma, 269
McArdle disease, 142
MDRD equation, 13
Medullary sponge kidney, 91
Melamine, 114
Membranoproliferative glomerulonephritis, 73
Membranous glomerulonephritis (MN), 211
Membranous nephropathy, 73
Mercury, 114
Mesangial cells, 197
Mesangiocapillary glomerulonephritis, 73
Metformin, 112–113
MGRS. *See* Monoclonal protein of renal
        significance (MGRS)
MGUS. *See* Monoclonal protein of
        undetermined significance (MGUS)
Microalbuminuria, 145
Microangiopathic haemolytic anaemia
        (MAHA), 177
Micturating cystogram, 96
MINT cocktail, 108, 112
Mitrofanoff fistula, 96
MN. *See* Membranous glomerulonephritis (MN)
Monoclonal protein of renal significance
        (MGRS), 199
Monoclonal protein of undetermined
        significance (MGUS), 199
Mononeuritis multiplex, 205
Multidisciplinary team, 243
Multiple myeloma, 190, 198
Mushrooms
    Chanterelle, 114
    Cortinarius species, 114
    Deadly Webcap, 114
    poisoning, 114
Myoglobinuria, 135, 140

N
Natural process limits, 35
Nephrin, 85
Nephritic syndrome, 202–205, 210
Nephritis, 134
Nephrocalcinosis, 88, 90
Nephrogenic systemic fibrosis (NSF), 229
Nephronophthisis, 92
Nephrotic-range proteinuria, 145
Nephrotic syndrome, 64, 74, 120, 149, 163,
        177, 198, 201, 202, 211
    minimal change, 151
Neutrophil Extracellular Traps (NETs), 206
NH_4^+. *See* Ammonium ions (NH_4^+)
Nitrites, 154
Nocturnal dipping, 126
Non-steroidal anti-inflammatory drugs
        (NSAIDs), 107
NSF. *See* Nephrogenic systemic fibrosis (NSF)

O
Obesity, 123
Oedema, 162
Oliguria, 164
Omeprazole, 112
Orellanine, 114
Oxygen sensing, 174

P
Papillary, necrosis, 177
Parathyroidectomy, 186
Parathyroid hormone (PTH), 182
Paroxysmal nocturnal haemoglobinuria
        (PNH), 177
PCR. *See* Protein:creatinine ratio (PCR)
Penicillin, 112
Peripheral neuropathy, 55
Peritoneal dialysis, 249, 262
PHD enzymes. *See* Prolyl-4-hydroxylase
        domain (PHD) enzymes
Phenolphthalein, 135
Phosphate, 181
Phosphatonins, 183
Pneumocystis jiroveci pneumonia (PJP), 267
PNH. *See* Paroxysmal nocturnal
        haemoglobinuria (PNH)
Podocin, 85
Podocyte, 150
Polycystic kidney disease:autosomal dominant
        (ADPKD), 91, 219
Polycystic kidney disease:autosomal
        recessive, 92

Polycystin, 92
Porphyria, 135
Post-streptococcal glomerulonephritis, 203, 204
Post-transplant lymphoproliferative disease (PTLD), 269
Postural hypotension, 201
Pre-eclampsia, 78–80
Pregabalin, 52, 53
Primary cilium, 92
Principal cells, 89
Prior odds, 197
Probability, 197
Prolyl-4-hydroxylase domain (PHD) enzymes, 174
Prostaglandins, 107
Protein:creatinine ratio (PCR), 145
Protein electrophoresis, 198
Proteinuria, 78, 129, 231, 237, 241
Proteus mirabilis, 154
Proton pump inhibitors, 112
Proximal tubule, 86
Pseudohypoaldosteronism:type 1 (PHA1), 89
Pseudohypoaldosteronism:type 2 (PHA2), 89
Psychosocial factors, 250
PTH. *See* Parathyroid hormone (PTH)
Purpura, 168
Pyruvate dehydrogenase, 113

R
Radio-contrast medium, 227
Recirculation, 259
Reference Change Value, 34
Reflux nephropathy, 96
Register, 276
Renal artery stenosis, 67–70
    flash pulmonary oedema, 67
Renal glycosuria, 88
Renal osteodystrophy, 184
Renal replacement therapy (RRT), 249
Renal tubular acidosis
    distal, 90
    proximal, 88
Renovascular disease, 170
Restless legs, 52
Retrograde ejaculation, 143
Retrograde urogram, 225
Retroperitoneal fibrosis, 220
Rhabdomyolysis, 113
Rickets
    hypophosphataemic, 88
    Vitamin D resistant, 88
Rifampicin, 135
Risk of death, 237

S
Salt intake, 163
Sarcoidosis, 190
Schwarz equation, 15
Seizures, 55
Sepsis syndrome, 164
Serum amyloid A protein, 73
Sexual intercourse, 154
Sickle cell anaemia, 177
Sir William Osler, 31
SLE. *See* Systemic lupus erythematosus (SLE)
Slit diaphragm, 150
Sodium bicarbonate, 181
Special cause, 35
Squamous cell carcinoma, 273
Stable, 35
Stages of CKD, 51–52
Statins, 142
Statistical Process Control (SPC), 35
Steal syndrome, 257
Stones, 154, 227
    calcium oxalate, 227
    cystine, 227
    magnesium ammonium phosphate, 227
    matrix stones, 227
    struvite, 227
Striped fibrosis, 108
'Surprise' question, 243
Surrogate endpoint, 145
Systemic lupus erythematosus (SLE), 198, 202, 203

T
Tacrolimus, 108
Tamm-Horsfall protein, 90, 135, 145
Target weight, 265
Technetium 99m dimercaptosuccinic acid (DMSA), 223
Technetium-99m mercaptoacetyltriglycine (MAG3), 223
Teratogenicity, 77
Thin glomerular basement membrane disease, 136
    nephropathy, 84
Thrombospondin type-1 domain-containing 7A (THSD7A), 211
Thrombotic thrombocytopaenic purpura (TTP), 79
Thrombotic thrombocytopenic purpura-hemolytic uremic syndrome (TTP-HUS), 179

THSD7A. *See* Thrombospondin type-1
    domain-containing 7A (THSD7A)
Total CO_2, 180
Transitional care, 123
Transplant, 249, 277
    rejection, 266
Treatment planning, 237
Trimethoprim, 25
TTP-HUS. *See* Thrombotic thrombocytopenic
    purpura-hemolytic uremic
    syndrome (TTP-HUS)
Tuberous sclerosis, 94
Tubule:collecting duct, 89–90
Tubule:distal, 87, 89
Tubulo-glomerular feedback, 112
Tubulotoxicity, 110–112

U
Ultrasound, 215
Uraemia
    pericarditis, 55
    pruritus, 52
Urea Reduction Ratio (URR), 55
Urea-to-creatinine ratio, 26, 105, 164
Ureteric obstruction, 129
Urethral stricture, 219

Urinary catheter, 153
Urinary infection, 96
Urine infection, 152
Uromodulin, 90, 135, 142, 145
    UMOD gene, 90
Uveitis, 205

V
Vasculitic illness, 205
Vasculitis, 167
Vasopressin, 89, 110
Verocytotoxin, 177
Vesicocolic fistula, 143
Vesicoureteric reflux, 78, 83, 95, 152
Vitamin D, 182
Vitamin D-binding protein (DBP), 184
Von-Hippel-Lindau disease, 94
Von Willebrand factor, 179

W
Warts, 270
Weight, 117
White coat effect, 125
Wilms-tumor-aniridia syndrome, 94

Printed by Printforce, the Netherlands